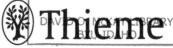

Supplement to NANDA International Nursing Diagnoses: Definitions and Classification, 2018–2020 (11th Edition)

New things you need to know

T. Heather Herdman, PhD, RN, FNI
Chief Executive Officer of NANDA International, Inc., Associate Professor, The University of Wisconsin-Green Bay, USA. Member of NANDA International since 1988, Diagnosis Development Committee Chair (1998–2004), President (2006–2008). Editor of *NANDA International Nursing Diagnoses: Definitions and Classification, 2009–2011*; Coeditor of *NANDA International Nursing Diagnoses: Definitions and Classification, 2015–2017* and *2018–2020.*

Shigemi Kamitsuru, PhD, RN, FNI
President of NANDA International, Inc., Nursing Diagnosis Consultant, Tokyo, Japan. Member of NANDA International since 1993, Diagnosis Development Committee Chair (2008–2012), President (2016–2020). Coeditor of *NANDA International Nursing Diagnoses: Definitions and Classification, 2015–2017 and 2018–2020.*

52 illustrations

Thieme
New York • Stuttgart • Delhi • Rio de Janeiro

Acquisitions Editor: Sue Hodgson
Managing Editor: Arindam Banerjee
Director, Editorial Services: Mary Jo Casey
Production Editor: Rohit Bhardwaj
International Production Director:
Andreas Schabert
Editorial Director: Sue Hodgson
International Marketing Director:
Fiona Henderson
International Sales Director: Louisa Turrell
Senior Vice President and Chief Operating
Officer: Sarah Vanderbilt
President: Brian D. Scanlan

Library of Congress Cataloging-in-Publication
Data is available from the publisher

© 2019 Thieme Medical Publishers, Inc.
Thieme Publishers New York
333 Seventh Avenue, New York, NY 10001 USA
+1 800 782 3488, customerservice@thieme.com

Thieme Publishers Stuttgart
Rüdigerstrasse 14, 70469 Stuttgart, Germany
+49 [0]711 8931 421, customerservice@thieme.de

Thieme Publishers Delhi
A-12, Second Floor, Sector-2, Noida-201301
Uttar Pradesh, India
+91 120 45 566 00, customerservice@thieme.in

Thieme Publishers Rio de Janeiro,
Thieme Publicações Ltda.
Edifício Rodolpho de Paoli, 25º andar
Av. Nilo Peçanha, 50 – Sala 2508
Rio de Janeiro 20020-906 Brasil
+55 21 3172 2297

Cover design: Thieme Publishing Group   54321
Typesetting by DiTech Process Solutions, India

Printed in USA by King Printing Company, Inc.

ISBN 978-1-68420-205-8

Also available as an e-book:
eISBN 978-1-68420-206-5

Important note: Medicine is an ever-changing science undergoing continual development. Research and clinical experience are continually expanding our knowledge, in particular our knowledge of proper treatment and drug therapy. Insofar as this book mentions any dosage or application, readers may rest assured that the authors, editors, and publishers have made every effort to ensure that such references are in accordance with **the state of knowledge at the time of production of the book.**

Nevertheless, this does not involve, imply, or express any guarantee or responsibility on the part of the publishers in respect to any dosage instructions and forms of applications stated in the book. **Every user is requested to examine carefully** the manufacturers' leaflets accompanying each drug and to check, if necessary in consultation with a physician or specialist, whether the dosage schedules mentioned therein or the contraindications stated by the manufacturers differ from the statements made in the present book. Such examination is particularly important with drugs that are either rarely used or have been newly released on the market. Every dosage schedule or every form of application used is entirely at the user's own risk and responsibility. The authors and publishers request every user to report to the publishers any discrepancies or inaccuracies noticed. If errors in this work are found after publication, errata will be posted at www.thieme.com on the product description page.

Some of the product names, patents, and registered designs referred to in this book are in fact registered trademarks or proprietary names even though specific reference to this fact is not always made in the text. Therefore, the appearance of a name without designation as proprietary is not to be construed as a representation by the publisher that it is in the public domain.

FSC
www.fsc.org
100%
Paper from well-managed forests
FSC® C103101

Contents

Preface

In this supplement to the 11th edition of the NANDA International, Inc., *NANDA International Nursing Diagnoses: Definitions and Classification, 2018–2020*, or the (NANDA-I) core text, many additions, revisions, and refinements have been introduced. The extent of these modifications is a testament to the continued evolution of nursing knowledge and NANDA-I's improved representation of that knowledge within the nursing diagnosis terminology.

Readers may please take note that this companion book is not written to be the primary text for those readers who are new to nursing diagnosis. They should read the core text, which includes chapters on the basics of diagnosis, assessment, clinical reasoning, and a solid introduction to the NANDA-I taxonomy. This companion book is designed to give current users of nursing diagnosis a "quick glance" into what is new in the 11th edition, as well as more in-depth information on some of those changes, including new diagnoses. In addition, conceptual issues that we believe require additional clarification in the upcoming 12th edition will be discussed, and some recommendations will be made for modification as the terminology continues to move forward.

We hope that you will find this book helpful as you use nursing diagnosis in your daily practice.

1 What is New?

As in the previous version, in this chapter you will find the addition of new **nursing** diagnoses, revisions to existing diagnoses, and removal of diagnoses from the terminology due to an unsatisfactory level of evidence. In addition, we will provide more detailed explanation about the two new categories of assessment data: *at-risk populations* and *associated conditions*. All of these modifications are introduced in the *NANDA-I Nursing Diagnoses: Definitions and Classification, 2018–2020* textbook. However, the purpose of this companion book is to provide more in-depth information to improve your understanding, to support education, and to facilitate implementation of these changes in practice.

Changes in the Overall Definition of Health Promotion Nursing Diagnosis

☞ *NANDA International Nursing Diagnoses: Definitions and Classification, 2018–2020,* p. 6

During this cycle of nursing diagnosis submission to the Diagnosis Development Committee (DCC), health promotion nursing diagnoses for the neonatal populations were reviewed. This led to discussion about the definition of health promotion diagnoses, which stated that the patient must "verbalize desire" for health promotion.

It was widely agreed that there are patients who are unable to verbalize (e.g., neonates, unconscious, comatose) but for whom health promotion is certainly a possibility, and that the nurse can act as an agent on behalf of those patients to promote health and well-being. Thus, the definition of health promotion nursing diagnosis was changed ▶ **Table 1-1.**

▶ **Table 1-1** Change to definition of health promotion nursing diagnosis

2015–2017 (10th edition)	2018–2020 (11th edition)
A clinical judgment concerning motivation and desire to increase well-being and to actualize health potential. These responses are expressed by a readiness to enhance specific health behaviors, and can be used in any health state. Health promotion responses may exist in an individual, family, group, or community	A clinical judgment concerning motivation and desire to increase well-being and to actualize health potential. These responses are expressed by a readiness to enhance specific health behaviors, and can be used in any health state. *In individuals who are unable to express their own readiness to enhance health behaviors, the nurse may determine that a condition for health promotion exists, and act on the client's behalf.* Health promotion responses may exist in an individual, family, group, or community

For example, the nursing diagnosis, *readiness for enhanced comfort* (00183) could be applicable for unconscious patients; likewise, the diagnosis, *readiness for enhanced organized infant behavior* (00117), is applicable to infants in the neonatal intensive care environment. Of note, this diagnosis has been slotted within the NANDA-I taxonomy for many years. As you can see from defining characteristics, which all began with the phrase "Parent expresses …," it was not conceptualized from the perspective of the infant, but from that of the parent's desire to enhance organized behavior of the infant. By changing the definition, the nurse can also act as an agent on behalf of the infant to promote health and well-being.

Changes to the Definitions Used for Risk Diagnoses

Although this is not indicated in the text, NANDA-I Nursing Diagnoses: Definitions and Classification, 2018–2020, users will notice a change in definitions of all risk diagnoses. Previously, we used the phrase, "Vulnerable to …" when beginning all definitions of risk diagnoses. In the current edition, this has been changed to read, "Susceptible to …". It was felt that this phrase was less judgmental, as the word "vulnerable" can infer helplessness rather than "at risk."

Introducing New Categories of Supportive Data for Diagnosis

An issue that has always been difficult for nurses to grasp is that of related factors and risk factors, as they have been described by NANDA-I.

Related factors are defined as: "Factors that appear to show some type of patterned relationship with the nursing diagnosis. Such factors may be described as antecedent to, associated with, related to, contributing to, or abetting."

☞ *NANDA International Nursing Diagnoses: Definitions and Classification, 2018–2020,* p. 137

And risk factors are defined as: "Environmental factors and physiological, psychological, genetic, or chemical elements that increase the vulnerability of an individual, family, group, or community to an unhealthy event."

☞ *NANDA International Nursing Diagnoses: Definitions and Classification, 2018–2020,* p. 137

As the terminology of NANDA-I has evolved over the years, so has our thinking. Originally, diagnoses included many factors that were felt to be helpful to clinical reasoning, even if it was a factor that could not be influenced by care provided. However, developers of NANDA-I have long taught that "whenever possible, nursing interventions should be aimed at these etiological factors in order to remove the underlying cause of the nursing diagnosis" (*NANDA International Nursing Diagnoses: Definitions and Classification, 2018–2020*, p. 39). Likewise, to prevent the risk nursing diagnosis, we have emphasized that nursing interventions should be aimed at those factors that increase the susceptibility. In reviewing the related factors and risk factors, there are many factors that are not amenable to independent nursing intervention. This has caused much confusion among students and bedside nurses over the years.

After much review and discussion, it was determined that many of the factors that had been categorized as "related factors" and "risk factors" were important for clinical reasoning, but nursing intervention could not remove or change them. To be clinicallyuseful and meet the goal of identifying etiological factors that can be removed or improved by nursing intervention, this needed to change.

It became apparent, after study, that these factors could be grouped into two categories: *at-risk populations* and *associated conditions*. Therefore, the lists of related factors and risk factors were reviewed and only those factors that could be removed or improved by nursing intervention were retained. The remaining factors, while considered supportive for clinical reasoning, were sorted into new categories, which we will now discuss in more detail.

It is important to note here that every country or geographical region specifies what interventions nurses can and cannot do within the scope of licensure. Therefore, as an international taxonomy, NANDA-I does its best to consider the scope of intervention found within the literature that reflects nursing practice on a global level. Obviously, there are some nurse practice laws and regulations that provide more autonomy for nurses and some that provide less. It is the responsibility of every professional nurse to be aware of the regulations where he/she practices, and to avoid interventions that would not be acceptable practice. Therefore, some nurses might say, "I can treat this NANDA-I associated condition in my practice," while others may say "I cannot treat this NANDA-I related factor." In some countries, nurses provide a great deal of intervention under a medical protocol, whereas in other countries nurses may not be able to provide certain interventions. We recognize that for some nurses, these data may seem "out of place," and refer you to your own regulations and scope of practice.

Finally, it should be noted that the recategorization of related factors and risk factors into these two new categories, for all diagnoses, was a significant piece of work. However, there was not sufficient time to enable revisions to those terms in the 10th edition. For example, "economically disadvantaged" can be found under the new category *at-risk populations* in more than 20 nursing diagnoses. To indicate it as a population, it would be better to state as "economically disadvantaged people" or "economically disadvantaged family." However, this 11th edition kept those expressions from the 10th version as they were. It is not a matter of merely changing the expression, but significant conceptual work is required. This work needs to be completed during this upcoming cycle so that the terms are more clinically useful.

At-risk Populations

One set of factors that was apparent included characteristics that could not be changed, either because they were demographic in nature (e.g., age, gender) or because they had occurred in the past (family or individual health history). These data were labeled as "at-risk populations" and are defined as:

Groups of people who share a characteristic that causes each member to be susceptible to a particular human response, such as demographics, health/ family history, stages of growth/development, or exposure to certain events/ experiences.

☞ NANDA International Nursing Diagnoses: Definitions and Classification, 2018–2020, p. 23–24

Rather than removing these terms completely from the terminology, it was determined to retain the data because they are helpful for nurses when considering diagnoses. If we know, for example, that *"women"* and those *"> 70 years of age"* are more likely to suffer from *frail elderly syndrome* (00257), that is important for us to consider, even though we cannot do anything to remove those susceptibilities for our patients. Similarly, if we know that *"age ≤ 2 years"* toddlers and *"age ≥ 65 years"* elderly are at higher *risk for falls* (00155), we would immediately determine the appropriateness of the diagnosis. Based on this diagnostic judgement, we are more attuned to the environment around those patients in an effort to prevent them from falling.

Associated Conditions

The other set of data that was apparent included characteristics that represent conditions that have been diagnosed by another health care professional, and/or forms of treatment that the patient may be receiving for these conditions. These data were therefore labeled as "associated conditions," and are defined as:

Medical diagnoses, injuries, procedures, medical devices, or pharmaceutical agents. These conditions are not independently modifiable by the professional nurse, but may support accuracy in nursing diagnosis.

☞ NANDA International Nursing Diagnoses: Definitions and Classification, 2018–2020, p. 24

If we know that a patient has the medical diagnosis, congestive heart failure *(circulatory problem)*, we would consider the influence of that general condition on the patient's daily life. Therefore, we would examine closely diagnoses of *activity intolerance* (00092) and *risk for activity intolerance* (00094), for example. However, our interventions cannot remove the congestive heart failure itself. Likewise, it is important for us to consider what medications (*pharmaceutical agent*) a patient is receiving and how those might affect his care and human responses, but we are not able to change the prescribed medications without an order from a health care provider who has prescriptive authority within each country.

Alignment of Diagnostic Indicators: Related Factors and Risk Factors

☞ *NANDA International Nursing Diagnoses: Definitions and Classification, 2018–2020,* p. 123

A review of concepts that include the same focus in problem-focused nursing diagnoses and risk nursing diagnoses (e.g., *caregiver roles strain* [00061], and *risk for caregiver role strain* [00062]) led to the recognition that there were discrepancies in diagnostic indicators. NANDA-I developers have always stated that there should be strong similarities between related factors for a problem-focused diagnosis and the risk factors for the risk diagnosis related to the same concept. In many cases, these factors could be identical, because the condition that puts you at risk for an undesirable response would most often be an etiology of that response should it occur.

For example, "*insufficient fiber intake*" and "*insufficient fluid intake*" are listed as related factors of *constipation* (00011). These factors also increase the vulnerability of the patient to constipation, that is, *risk for constipation* (00015). In both cases, nursing interventions should be available to decrease the unfavorable response or modify its risk of occurrence.

Therefore, users will notice that related factors of the problem-focused nursing diagnoses, and risk factors of the risk nursing diagnoses, are now identical or nearly identical in the 11th edition. We used the following process to align related factors and risk factors:
- Combined all related factors and risk factors
- Removed one of the factors in case of overlap
- Standardized terms of a factor that had the same meaning but different expressions
- Categorized factors into related/risk factors, at-risk population, and associated condition

When the expressions of related factors and risk factors were slightly different and we were unable to determine whether to standardize the terms, tentatively, we left two terms as they are. That is why you may sometimes find two very similar factors in related/risk factors.

However, because this first step was to align the current lists of diagnostic indicators, it should be noted that in many cases, conceptual work is needed to ensure these are the most evidence-based indicators for these diagnoses.

Seventeen New Nursing Diagnoses

☞ *NANDA International Nursing Diagnoses: Definitions and Classification, 2018–2020,* p. 7–9

There were 17 new nursing diagnoses in this edition:
- Readiness for enhanced health literacy (00262)
- Ineffective adolescent eating dynamics (00269)
- Ineffective child eating dynamics (00270)
- Ineffective infant feeding dynamics (00271)
- Risk for metabolic imbalance syndrome (00263)
- Imbalanced energy field (00273)
- Risk for unstable blood pressure (00267)
- Risk for complicated immigration transition (00260)
- Acute substance withdrawal syndrome (00258)
- Risk for acute substance withdrawal syndrome (00259)
- Neonatal abstinence syndrome (00264)
- Risk for surgical site infection (00266)
- Risk for dry mouth (00261)
- Risk for venous thromboembolism (00268)
- Risk for female genital mutilation (00272)
- Risk for occupational injury (00265)
- Risk for ineffective thermoregulation (00274)

These will be discussed in detail in chapter 4, with model case studies, general outcomes, and nursing interventions.

Revisions to 11 Nursing Diagnosis Labels

☞ *NANDA International Nursing Diagnoses: Definitions and Classification, 2018–2020,* p. 9, 21

Changes were made to 11 nursing diagnosis labels, as seen in ▶ **Table1-2-1-6**. Some background was provided on pages 9 and 21 of the core NANDA-I textbook; however, here we will provide some more detailed explanation.

The reason for the change in ▸ **Table 1-2** was due to the lack of an identified human response within the label. As it was originally written, the condition, "*deficient diversional activity*," could result merely from a lack of activities available in an organization/institution where the patient is receiving care. "*Deficient diversional activity*" is perhaps a cause or a symptom of a human response, but when we change the term to "*decreased diversional activity engagement*," we are now talking about how the individual responds to a reduction in recreational or leisure activities.

Similarly, "*insufficient breast milk*" may be a symptom of an underlying problem, but when our focus changes to "*insufficient breast milk production*," we are now looking at a physiological human response (which may be influenced by internal and external factors).

Finally, "*impaired oral mucous membrane*" is also a symptom, or a statement of the location of a symptom, but when we shift the focus to "*impaired oral mucous membrane integrity*," we are now considering a physiological human response. With "integrity" representing the human response in the label, nurses are directed to assess and treat integrity of the mucous membranes as well as that of tissue and of skin.

The rationale for the change in ▸ **Table 1-3** is that jaundice—the yellow discoloration of skin and mucous membranes—is merely one symptom of the underlying response. Nurses in many countries independently diagnose and treat these conditions, so it was felt appropriate to include these diagnoses within the terminology, but with a change in focus to represent the real issue of the concern "hyperbilirubinemia."

In the instance in ▸ **Table 1-4**, the use of the term "syndrome" in the label is not appropriate. "Risk for sudden infant death syndrome" suggests that the infant is at risk for the syndrome itself; however, the risk which a nurse has to prevent is

▸Table 1-2 Changes to nursing diagnosis labels

2015–2017 (10th edition)	2018–2020 (11th edition)
Deficient diversional activity (00097)	Decreased diversional activity engagement
Insufficient breast milk (00216)	Insufficient breast milk production
Impaired oral mucous membrane (00045)	Impaired oral mucous membrane integrity
Risk for impaired oral mucous membrane (00247)	Risk for impaired oral mucous membrane integrity

▸Table 1-3 Changes to nursing diagnosis labels

2015–2017 (10th edition)	2018–2020 (11th edition)
Neonatal jaundice (00194)	Neonatal hyperbilirubinemia
Risk for neonatal jaundice (00230)	Risk for neonatal hyperbilirubinemia

▶**Table 1-4** Changes to nursing diagnosis labels

2015–2017 (10th edition)	2018–2020 (11th edition)
Risk for sudden infant death syndrome (00156)	Risk for sudden infant death

in fact "sudden death." Moreover, "sudden infant death syndrome" is not diagnosed until after the baby's death.

The change in ▶**Table1-5** was to add specificity to the response of concern; "trauma" could relate to physical, psychological, or spiritual trauma.

Rationale for these changes in ▶**Table1-6** was to be consistent with the literature which refers to this diagnosis as a "reaction" rather than a "response."

NANDA-I is constantly reviewing the terminology to improve the consistency within the terms. If you notice additional areas of inconsistency between terms, we would encourage you to provide feedback for the DCC. Contact information is available on the NANDA-I website (www.nanda.org).

▶**Table 1-5** Changes to nursing diagnosis labels

2015–2017 (10th edition)	2018–2020 (11th edition)
Risk for trauma (00038)	Risk for physical trauma

▶**Table 1-6** Changes to nursing diagnosis labels

2015–2017 (10th edition)	2018–2020 (11th edition)
Risk for allergy response (00217)	Risk for allergy reaction
Latex allergy response (00041)	Latex allergy reaction
Risk for latex allergy response (00042)	Risk for latex allergy reaction

Revisions to 72 Nursing Diagnoses

☞ *NANDA International Nursing Diagnoses: Definitions and Classification, 2018–2020,* p. 7, 10–20

Seventy-two diagnoses were revised during this cycle.

Please see the *NANDA International Nursing Diagnoses: Definitions and Classification, 2018–2020* textbook for revised definitions and diagnostic indicators (defining characteristics, related factors, and risk factors) and submitters. ▶**Table 3.2** in that book (p. 10–20) identifies all revisions that were made.

All literature references that were used as evidence to support the submission of these diagnoses are available from the website, www.MediaCenter.

Thieme.com. Please note that you need to enter the specific code found in the front cover of the book.

Eight Nursing Diagnoses Removed from Taxonomy II

☞ *NANDA International Nursing Diagnoses: Definitions and Classification, 2018–2020,* p. 7, 9

Eight nursing diagnoses were removed from the taxonomy:
- Noncompliance (00079)
- Readiness for enhanced fluid balance (00160)
- Readiness for enhanced urinary elimination (00166)
- Risk for impaired cardiovascular function (00239)
- Risk for ineffective gastrointestinal perfusion (00202)
- Risk for ineffective renal perfusion (00203)
- Risk for imbalanced body temperature (00005)
- Risk for disproportionate growth (00113)

The first six of these diagnoses were removed, after the DCC reviewed them, because they were inconsistent with current literature, or lacked sufficient evidence to support their continuation within the terminology. For example, the diagnosis of *noncompliance* is no longer consistent with current literature that addresses this response as *nonadherence*. Further, the concept of compliance is far more judgmental and paternalistic than that of adherence, which has been adopted as we have adopted a more patient-focused philosophy of care. *Risk for ineffective renal perfusion* was removed because, after careful consideration by the DDC members, it was determined that independent nursing intervention could not prevent a decrease in blood circulation to the kidney, as evidenced by risk factors representing medical diagnoses.

The seventh diagnosis, *risk for imbalanced body temperature* was replaced by a new diagnosis, *risk for ineffective thermoregulation* (00274). Revisions to this diagnosis led to the recognition that the concept of interest was "thermoregulation," rather than "body temperature," and the definition and risk factors were consistent with the existing diagnosis, *ineffective thermoregulation* (00008). Changing the label (focus of diagnosis) and the definition was more substantial than a diagnosis revision, so the original diagnosis was retired, and a new diagnosis was submitted.

The eighth diagnosis, *risk for disproportionate growth* was removed because it contained two different populations of concern, with different underlying etiologies, within its definition (> 97th or < 3rd percentile for age). In the 2015–2017 edition, it was indicated to retire from the NANDA-I taxonomy unless additional work is completed to separate the focus, but no work was submitted. We hope that pediatric nurses will develop and submit diagnoses for both of these populations.

Diagnostic Indicator Terms Were Standardized

☞ *NANDA International Nursing Diagnoses: Definitions and Classification, 2018–2020,* p. 21–23

Examples used to explain defining characteristics, related factors, or risk factors have been removed. The purpose of the examples was to clarify intent; however, some appeared to be more accurately representing "teaching tips," and those have been removed. Abbreviations were also removed from all diagnostic indicator terms.

When the same diagnostic indicator term lists different examples, it was problematic in standardizing terms. For instance, examples of a related factor, "*environmental barrier*," in *insomnia* (00095) lists: ambient noise, daylight/darkness exposure, ambient temperature/humidity, unfamiliar setting, and in *impaired transfer ability* (00090) lists: bed height, inadequate space, wheelchair type, treatment equipment, restraints.

In the 2018–2020 edition, both diagnoses have a related factor "*environmental barrier*" without examples. It is acknowledged that some of the terms used for diagnostic indicators may be vague or require additional clarification to improve clinical usefulness. What is important in standardizing terms is a definition. The common definition guarantees that nurses can use the term anytime and anywhere in the same way. Given this perspective, as each NANDA-I nursing diagnosis has definition, we may need definitions for diagnostic indicator terms. However, this is no easy task because there are over 3,500 such terms.

It is recommended that users suggest ways to improve these terms to NANDA-I, to make them more useful.

Did NANDA-I Approve Taxonomy III?

☞ *NANDA International Nursing Diagnoses: Definitions and Classification, 2018–2020,* p. 86–87

A proposed change to the NANDA-I taxonomy III was published in the 10th edition of the NANDA-I textbook (pp. 81–90, ▶ **Table 3.2**). The membership, in 2016, voted on whether to adopt taxonomy III, and by an overwhelming majority, the decision was to remain with taxonomy II. Therefore, there is no change to the NANDA-I taxonomic structure.

2 Issues and Upcoming Activities

In the last version of this book, we discussed many issues within the NANDA-I taxonomy. While some of these were resolved this cycle, others remain and will require work over the coming years.

The evolution of our scientific language is a continual process; there is no "end point" at which the terminology will be "complete." Rather, there will be continued revisions, removals from, and additions to the terminology as knowledge evolves. Likewise, there are ways to better position the NANDA-I terminology as the strongest, evidence-based, and standardized nursing diagnostic language. Some of these evolutions are more editorial in nature, such as developing a specific schema for definitions and structure of diagnostic indicator terms. Others are more involved, and we will discuss each of these below.

What is the Evidence Base for Current Nursing Diagnoses?

Nursing should be an evidence-based science and, as such, requires evidence to support our diagnoses. It is critical that we are able to identify clinical studies that validate nursing diagnoses across populations, cultures, and settings. If differences between the current taxonomy and the clinical study findings are noted, these need to be identified within the taxonomy to ensure support for clinical reasoning.

Many of our current diagnoses are slotted at the lowest level of evidence (LOE) allowed for entry into the taxonomy (2.1). It is believed that, in many cases, these diagnoses actually have significant research findings that would support a higher LOE, but that this work has not been collected and submitted to change this for the diagnoses. We look forward to the efforts of nurses interested in such research.

We also have numerous diagnoses that were accepted into the taxonomy prior to initiation of LOE criteria, and these require review to determine their LOE status. You might have noticed the following footnote in some diagnoses: *This diagnosis will retire from the NANDA-I taxonomy in the 2021–2023 edition unless additional work is completed to bring it up to a level of evidence 2.1 or higher.* We hope many readers understand the current situation and work with us to advance nursing diagnosis research.

In addition, there are concerns about the appropriateness of the current LOE criteria. Therefore, a new LOE criteria has been proposed by a task force appointed by the Research and Education Committee which will be reviewed in the upcoming cycle.

Can a Symptom be a Nursing Diagnosis?

Although the terminology has accepted a multiaxial system, some of the current diagnoses do not fit within this system. They may, in actuality, be the symptoms: *nausea* (00134), *constipation* (00011), *insomnia* (00095), *fatigue* (00093), *anxiety* (00146), *fear* (00148), *helplessness* (00124), etc. Is the human response we are diagnosing actually *anxiety* or is it the *ineffective management of anxiety*? What is the actual judgment about this symptom/response? Many people experience anxiety at times, and in fact this is a defense mechanism that human beings share; what is the level of anxiety at which this otherwise normal response becomes of concern to nursing?

Currently, we consider *insomnia* and *fear* to be nursing diagnoses, but they can be found as diagnostic indicator terms (defining characteristics/related factors/risk factors) within other nursing diagnoses. Nurses then ask, "Am I supposed to diagnose the *insomnia* itself, or should I consider it as a diagnostic indicator of another nursing diagnosis?" It is difficult to comprehend they can be both defining characteristics and diagnoses.

We recommend a review of this issue to determine whether or not symptoms belong within the NANDA-I nursing diagnosis taxonomy. Perhaps a secondary taxonomy of symptoms is needed within NANDA-I, or perhaps we need to determine that these symptoms do not fit within the multiaxial system, and remove them from the terminology altogether. Currently, symptom management is receiving a great deal of attention within the nursing literature. We need to reconceptualize symptoms that are found within the NANDA-I taxonomy to reflect this issue. For example, rather than using the diagnosis *nausea*, perhaps the response is *ineffective nausea management*, and rather than *acute pain*, perhaps the response is *ineffective pain management.* However, it would be important that these diagnoses would focus on the patient's response, and not an issue with nursing care, as the focus of nursing diagnosis is the patient's human response.

What is the Appropriate Level of Granularity for Nursing Diagnoses?

One frequent topic of discussion is what level of granularity should be used for diagnoses in the terminology. Should the diagnoses be broad, concrete, or both for clinical practice? Discussion of levels of granularity is important, because it will support the decision-making of nurses developing/revising diagnoses, and that of those individuals tasked with review of diagnosis submissions to the NANDA-I.

For example, in the new edition, two problem-focused diagnoses have been accepted that address issues with ineffective eating dynamics:
- Ineffective adolescent eating dynamics (00233)
- Ineffective child eating dynamics (00270)

These terms are very specifically diagnosed through assessment data that differ based on the age of the subject. However, there is no broad diagnosis that would address the problem of eating dynamics of all age groups, such as ineffective eating dynamics.

When we look at other foci of diagnoses, we can find different levels of granularity present in the terminology. For example, the diagnosis, *risk for injury* (00035) is broader than *risk for corneal injury* (00245) and *risk for urinary tract injury* (00250). Some nurses would argue that *risk for injury* (00035) is the only diagnosis required, because *corneal injury* and *urinary tract injury* could be prevented using this diagnosis; other nurses prefer the more concrete diagnoses. In general, however, more granular or more specific diagnoses may better direct specific patient care.

It is our belief that it is appropriate to have a variety of levels of granularity within the terminology. We believe that it is important to have more abstract (broader) terms, because they help us organize the terminology (to classify nursing diagnosis terms). Having the broader term may also support clinical reasoning by helping us categorize our thinking—you may, for example, notice *risk for infection* (00004) first, and then upon further assessment and/or reflection, narrow the focus to *risk for surgical site infection* (00266).

However, there might be value in determining what level of granularity would be considered sufficient. For example, considering the examples above, is there a level of granularity that might be considered too discrete? Would we want to have a diagnosis, for example, of *risk for toenail injury*?

What is Needed to Improve Translation?

The issue of granularity is also important in translation, in the understanding of the focus of the nursing diagnosis in different languages, and in the applicability in clinical practice internationally. An example of this might be the diagnosis, *risk for falls* (00155). A person can fall down the stairs, fall out of bed, or fall down while walking across the room. However, in the original English language, there is just this one word—"fall"—that is used to express any unintended drop from higher surfaces, or from the same surface. In many languages, this would not be expressed using the same word(s), and so the translation, understanding, and applicability of the original English terms may be difficult. It may be necessary to consider that some languages would be better served to have different nursing diagnosis labels to address those phenomena that cannot accurately be translated as one term from the original English language.

When translating a word from one language to another, it is often not a one-to-one replacement. For instance, the word "feeding" is included in some diagnoses, such as *feeding self-care deficit* (00102) and *ineffective infant feeding pattern* (00107). In English, the word "feeding" can mean: an instance of eating (e.g., "he is able to manage feeding activities"), or taking nourishment (e.g., "the infant is feeding well"), or providing nourishment (e.g., "the caregiver is feeding her client"). In all cases, the English word "feeding" is appropriate and conveys this variety of actions. However, in many languages, these are distinct actions that are discussed using different terms.

Thus, the translation from English into other languages can be confusing and may lack the full intent of the term. Back translation may be necessary to ensure that the words used in translation truly match the intent of the original language. Likewise, consideration should be given to determine if there are other words in the original language that would better describe the phenomena and that would be more easily translated.

Another consideration may be the use of a thesaurus of terms for translation and/or for those terms that are more culturally and clinically relevant. There may be examples in which a term used in English has no actual translation into other languages, and a detailed description is therefore required to facilitate understanding. Matching these descriptions to the original term in a thesaurus ensures that standardization of intent is maintained.

How Should a Nursing Diagnosis be Defined?

In the 10th and 11th editions, an attempt has been made to bring consistency to the different types of nursing diagnosis definitions. For example, risk and health promotion diagnoses were all changed to reflect similar patterns respectively. In this manner, risk diagnoses use the format, "susceptible to..., which may compromise health"; health promotion diagnosis definitions use the phrase "which can be strengthened."

However, some of the definitions of the nursing diagnoses are not particularly helpful to a nurse who is trying to understand the meaning of the diagnoses. For example, it might be helpful for a nurse to see, when looking at the definition of *ineffective health maintenance* (00099), that the focus of the diagnosis is "health maintenance," it is located in Class 2 (health management), under Domain 1 (health promotion), and how it is differentiated from other related diagnoses, such as *ineffective health management* (00078). This could be accomplished with an outline or mapping of where the concept is located within the taxonomy, along with the verbal description (definition) of the nursing diagnosis itself.

Additionally, some diagnoses adopt definitions that have been approved by national or international groups (e.g., the World Health Organization or the National Pressure Ulcer Advisory Panel, USA); in other diagnoses, a definition may be adopted from one particular research article, which is then cited as a reference for the definition; while in others, no particular quote or previously accepted definition is used. No standard currently exists as to when it is appropriate to use a previously accepted definition, when/if one should quote a single article's definition, or if all definitions should be developed specifically for the nursing diagnosis definition within the terminology. This issue should be further discussed, until the structure for a diagnosis definition is finalized.

Syndrome Nursing Diagnoses are Specific Clusters of Nursing Diagnoses

The definition for syndrome nursing diagnoses indicates that a syndrome represents a clinical judgment that describes a cluster of nursing diagnoses that occur together, and are best addressed together and through similar interventions. However, it has not been clearly identified whether or not defining characteristics can also include signs/symptoms that are not current nursing diagnoses. Therefore, syndrome diagnoses may currently include nursing diagnoses and other signs/symptoms. This can be confusing to the user, and should be clarified.

We recommend that work be undertaken to remove from the defining characteristics all signs/symptoms that are not represented as nursing diagnosis, or to consider ways to cluster these signs/symptoms together into nursing diagnoses. For example, in the defining characteristics of *relocation stress syndrome* (00114), there are two diagnoses, anxiety (00146) and fear (00148), but others are signs/symptoms. However, anxiety and fear are also symptoms as we explained previously. We need to examine whether "alteration in sleep pattern" is same as *sleep pattern disturbances* (00198), as well as "loss of self-worth" and "low self-esteem" can be replaced with *situational low self-esteem* (00120). All syndrome diagnoses that were developed prior to the 9th edition should be reviewed and revised to ensure congruence with the definition of syndrome diagnoses.

The other confusing issue for users is when a syndrome is included within a risk nursing diagnosis label. For example, *risk for metabolic imbalance syndrome* (00263) has seven nursing diagnoses listed as risk factors. These diagnoses are risk diagnoses, not syndromes. At present, there is no requirement that risk factors for these syndromes must be nursing diagnoses. The question remains, should the risk factors in fact be nursing diagnoses, or should they be individual symptoms?

Do We All Use Health Promotion Nursing Diagnoses in the Same Way?

Nursing diagnoses should be based on the condition, preference, and readiness of the patient, whenever possible. However, the 11th edition introduces a change to the definition, as we previously noted, that allows the nurse to act on behalf of nonverbal patients.

That said, consideration for the use of health promotion nursing diagnoses has often been based on the individual preference of the *nurse* rather than the patient. Nurses who are more focused on health promotion may gravitate toward these diagnoses, while those in more intensive care environments may gravitate toward problem-focused diagnoses or risk diagnoses. This brings to light the importance of discussing with patients their nursing diagnoses and allowing them to participate in the decision-making as to whether a diagnosis might be a health promotion diagnosis or a risk diagnosis, for example. Considering the patient's values and beliefs has always been an integral component of the nursing process and clinical reasoning, and this is an excellent way to encourage patient–nurse dialogue on areas of concern to the nurse.

Diagnosis of health promotion responses may be more difficult, in some ways, because the same clinical picture might be a problem-focused, risk or health promotion diagnosis: it is the context of the patient that enables the differentiation. The patient who recognizes opportunity to improve and wants to do so is a candidate for health promotion; the patient who does not recognize the need to change is not.

It is important to consider outcomes for health promotion diagnoses. Outcomes should not be based on a continuing desire to promote or enhance health, but on the issue of focus. For example, *readiness for enhanced parenting* (00164) should be evaluated based on demonstrated enhancements to the home environment and/or enhanced emotional support of children, etc. It is possible that, after a period of time, a reevaluation of this diagnosis may show no progress. Perhaps the parent verbalizes a desire to enhance her emotional support of her child, but has made no movement on doing so. It may become necessary to discontinue the health promotion diagnosis and convert to a risk, or problem-focused diagnosis, based on newer assessment data. Conversely, the risk diagnosis, *risk for impaired parenting* (00057), may convert to health promotion diagnosis when the parent has made good progress, and now states a desire to enhance parenting skills even further.

It might also be helpful to consider Prochaska's Transtheoretical Model, which discusses six stages of readiness for behavioral change. These stages are: precontemplation, contemplation, preparation, action, maintenance, and termination. Patients may not be ready to enhance particular behaviors if they are in precontemplation or contemplation phases, which could suggest that the use of health promotion diagnoses in these individuals who are not ready/motivated would not be effective, and perhaps a risk diagnosis or a problem-focused diagnosis would be more appropriate (http://www.pro-change.com/transtheoretical-model-of-behavior-change).

In the future, we would like to suggest that we evaluate how nurses can best identify when these diagnoses are most appropriate, to avoid a situation in which one nurse might address a diagnosis from a risk perspective, while her colleague chooses to address it from the health promotion perspective. The concern with this is we would lose the ability to track the response over time, if nurses are inconsistent in how they diagnose the human response due to personal philosophy rather than patient status, preference, or readiness. As we move into the electronic health record, this could limit our ability to collect data that provides insight into patient outcomes and effective interventions across the continuum of care, and/or over time.

Is There a Consistency Across Nursing Diagnoses That Share Common Foci?

There are many nursing diagnoses within the taxonomy that share a common focus. For example, there are several diagnoses related to coping, fluid volume, breastfeeding, parenting, and injury. It is critical, to avoid confusion, that those common foci are defined in the same manner. At this time, there are no standardized definitions of the foci of diagnoses, nor are there clear linkages between the foci of diagnoses and defined terms within the taxonomy.

Likewise, there has not been any emphasis on using the taxonomy itself as a structure for the development of diagnoses. There are definitions for domains and classes within the NANDA-I taxonomy, so when there are diagnoses that use the same terms, there should be an assured consistency between the definitions of the domain, class, and diagnosis. ▶**Table 2-1** shows definitions of terms related to coping in taxonomy II, but it is hard to find consistency.

▶Table 2-1 Definitions of domain, class, and nursing diagnoses related to coping

Terms related to coping	Definition
Domain 9 Coping/stress tolerance	Contending with life events/life processes
Class 2 Coping responses	The process of managing environmental stress
Defensive coping (00071)	Repeated projection of falsely positive self-evaluation based on a self-protective pattern that defends against underlying perceived threats to positive self-regard
Ineffective coping (00069)	A pattern of invalid appraisal of stressors, with cognitive and/or behavioral efforts, that fails to manage demands related to well-being
Readiness for enhanced coping (00158)	A pattern of valid appraisal of stressors with cognitive and/or behavioral efforts to manage demands related to well-being, which can be strengthened

(Continued)

►Table 2-1 (Continued)

Compromised family coping (00074)	A usually supportive primary person (family member, significant other, or close friend) provides insufficient, ineffective, or compromised support, comfort, assistance, or encouragement that may be needed by the client to manage or master adaptive tasks related to his or her health challenge
Ineffective community coping (00077)	A pattern of community activities for adaptation and problem-solving that is unsatisfactory for meeting the demands or needs of the community

Consistency in Use of NANDA-I Terms in Other Works

The purpose of standardization of a terminology is to ensure that all nurses can be confident that they understand one another when they communicate their judgments, through the use of the same terms. In other words, if all nurses understand the meaning of a term, such as *activity intolerance* (00092), they will define it in the same way, and use the same list of diagnostic indicators to validate their assessment of the phenomena in practice. When this occurs, there is a true standardization of terminology. If, however, nurses use the term, *activity intolerance*, but define the phenomena differently or validate it using a different list of indicators, how do we know what is really meant by that term?

To ensure standardization, and the safe use of a terminology, NANDA-I began requiring authors to use the exact nursing diagnosis label, definition and diagnostic indicators when using the terminology in their own works, beginning with the 9th edition. Authors who adapt, remove, or add to the terminology must clearly indicate what differs from the NANDA-I terms, as the previous lack of doing so has caused confusion in practice, education, and research.

What might appear to be a minor change can, in actuality, have significant implications on the meaning of a term. For example, consider the change of the word "or" to the word "and," in the following definition. *Ineffective breathing pattern* (00032) is defined as the "inspiration and/or expiration that does not provide adequate ventilation." A change in this definition to "inspiration AND expiration…" alters its meaning. Does this now apply to individuals with difficulty with inspiration alone? No, it would not.

Standardization of translations of terms is also a concern. It is important that terms are translated consistently throughout the terminology. Further, it is critical that as the NANDA-I content is used across other authors' works, the official language translations are always maintained in their entirety. Again, the purpose here is to avoid confusion and to ensure safety and accuracy in communication.

3 Clinical Reasoning Models

Clinical reasoning models position nursing diagnosis as the driving force in the nursing process by illustrating logical relationships among nursing diagnosis, outcomes, and nursing interventions. Once a nursing diagnosis is identified accurately, based on proper diagnostic indicators (defining characteristics, risk factors, and related factors), you will be amazed how simple it is to identify outcomes and select interventions. In Chapter 4, we use these models to identify general goals, outcomes, and nursing interventions for model cases of the 17 new nursing diagnoses.

Nursing Diagnosis Drives the Nursing Process

Without an accurate nursing diagnosis, it is not possible to identify proper nursing outcomes, to plan and implement effective nursing interventions, or to evaluate the progress toward the identified outcomes. In other words, accurate nursing diagnosis is the absolute requirement for the nursing process to flow smoothly. This leads to several questions. How can we identify a nursing diagnosis accurately? How should we identify expected outcomes? How should we select interventions that work for the particular patient?

There are some texts that indicate general relationships, which exist among the NANDA International (NANDA-I), Nursing Outcomes Classification (NOC), and Nursing Interventions Classification (NIC) (Johnson, et al., 2006) terms. However, it is not practical to review these texts for appropriate nursing outcomes and nursing interventions every time we develop a care plan for a nursing diagnosis we have identified. Furthermore, it may take several months, and in some cases several years, after a new edition of NANDA-I terminology is released for such books to be published. Nevertheless, some nurses think that new NANDA-I nursing diagnoses cannot be used until these predefined relationships are available. This is simply not accurate. If standardized language does not exist, or is not in use in one's organization, for outcomes or interventions, nurses must clearly document what they intend as an outcome and what interventions they are using to obtain that outcome. Further, each patient is unique and so what may be an obvious link in one patient will not make sense in another.

There are simple and logical relationships among a nursing diagnosis, outcomes, and nursing interventions. The Clinical Reasoning Model (Kamitsuru, 2009) shows these relationships clearly. A nursing diagnosis plays a role as the driving force of the nursing process. Therefore, once nursing diagnosis is determined, we simply need to apply basic rules to determine the rest.

The Clinical Reasoning Model was constructed using one of the theory development methods (Kim, 2003). Various authors' perspectives regarding the relationships among nursing diagnosis, nursing outcomes, and nursing interventions were reviewed and deductively synthesized to create the model. The model has been tested at multiple nursing diagnosis workshops, and its validity has been confirmed.

The Clinical Reasoning Model consists of three different submodels:
1. Clinical Reasoning Model I: problem-focused nursing diagnosis
2. Clinical Reasoning Model II: risk nursing diagnosis
3. Clinical Reasoning Model III: health promotion nursing diagnosis

Each model integrates four essential components of clinical reasoning in the nursing process: diagnostic reasoning, goal and outcome reasoning, nursing intervention reasoning, and evaluation reasoning.

Clinical Reasoning Model I: Problem-Focused Nursing Diagnosis

Let's start with the model for problem-focused nursing diagnoses (▶ **Fig. 3-1**). At first glance, the model may seem complicated. However, by breaking it down into its four components, it becomes quite simple to understand, and easy to apply in practice.

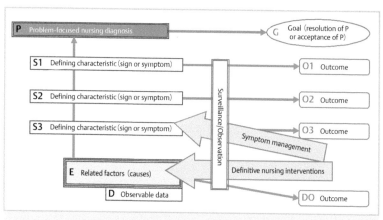

Fig. 3-1 Clinical Reasoning Model I: problem-focused nursing diagnosis

Problem-focused nursing diagnosis: diagnostic reasoning

▶ **Figure 3-2** shows the *diagnostic reasoning* component. The problem-focused nursing diagnosis consists of:
- P: the label of the nursing diagnosis, problem
- S: defining characteristics, signs and symptoms

- E: related factors, etiology, causes of the problem
- D: if the related factor term is too abstract, it may be helpful to clarify using actual observable data

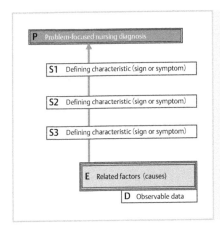

Fig. 3-2 Problem-focused nursing diagnosis: diagnostic reasoning

Signs are the objective data that the nurse collects through her senses. For example, a patient's skin may be dry, smooth, or rough to the touch. The breath sounds may be clear, or there may be rales. *Symptoms* are the subjective data of the patient, and what the nurse is told by the patient and/or his family/friends. For example, the patient may report that he is having trouble with his breathing, or having a sharp pain in his stomach. Signs and symptoms are categorized as *defining characteristics* in the NANDA-I taxonomy.

Related factors are basically those things that cause the diagnosis, and they need either to be modifiable or are able to be removed with independent nursing interventions.

To identify a problem-focused nursing diagnosis accurately, it is important to perform a thorough nursing assessment and identify data and information that support the diagnosis: the defining characteristics and related factors. Practically, these data and information are collected from the physical examination and interviews.

To identify defining characteristics and related factors to be used as the basis for the diagnosis, please refer to the text, *NANDA International Nursing Diagnoses: Definitions and Classification, 2018–2020*. However, some of the diagnoses have a long list of defining characteristics and related factors; and that may be confusing. In such a case, we advise you to review the meaning of the diagnosis by studying the definition, and to utilize your reasoning skills based on accumulated knowledge and experience.

Problem-focused nursing diagnosis: goal and outcome reasoning

The second part is the *goal and outcome reasoning* component (▶ **Fig. 3-3**). The goal (G) is at the top, and it is much broader than outcomes (O). The data outcome (DO) represented in the model is the outcome of the observable data of the related factors.

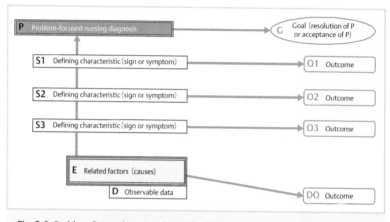

Fig. 3-3 Problem-focused nursing diagnosis: goal and outcome reasoning

A goal can be either the resolution of the problem, or acceptance of the problem. For most of the diagnoses, the goal is resolution of the problem. However, the complete resolution of a chronic problem is not possible, such as with *chronic pain* (00133). In this case, the realistic goal may be acceptance of the problem.

If we view the goal (G) to be the ultimate end-point of care, outcomes (O) could be seen as short-term goals or objectives to be achieved as we move toward the ultimate end-point of care. Outcomes are logically derived from the signs and symptoms: the defining characteristics. Likewise, outcomes of the related factors (causes) can be inferred as the resolution or modification of those factors.

For instance, the goal of the diagnosis, *disturbed sleep pattern* (00198) can be easily reasoned from the label; that is, *resolution of the disturbed sleep pattern* or *restoration of a good sleep pattern*. If defining characteristics are *difficulty initiating sleep, difficulty maintaining sleep state*, and *dissatisfaction with sleep*, then outcomes can be easily reasoned to be *ease in falling asleep, able to maintain sleep state*, and *increased satisfaction with sleep*.

Currently different terminologies, such as NOC, are used in conjunction with NANDA-I diagnoses. However, if we develop or adopt standardized scales, we can use them for assessment as well as for evaluation. For example, think about the nursing diagnosis of *impaired skin integrity* (00046). If the patient has destruction of the skin layers, and this is confirmed objectively using a standardized scale, then we can use that same scale not only for the daily assessment, but also for evaluating the progress of the skin condition toward identified outcomes. Development of such standardized scales are an urgent priority for the science of nursing diagnosis.

Problem-focused nursing diagnosis: nursing intervention reasoning

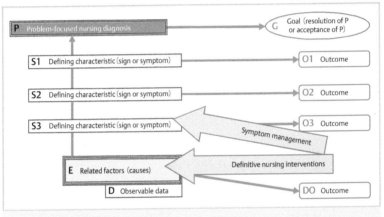

Fig. 3-4 Problem-focused nursing diagnosis: nursing intervention reasoning

Next is the *nursing intervention reasoning* component (▶ **Fig. 3-4**). There are two different arrows pointing from the goal/outcome component. The longer arrow pointing toward the related factors represents the definitive nursing interventions. The other arrow, pointing toward the defining characteristics, relates to symptom management.

Related factors are causes of the problem-focused nursing diagnosis. If we remove those causes by definitive nursing interventions, we can resolve the problem. When defining characteristics include a distressing symptom, symptom management becomes a part of the intervention. *Symptoms* can be treated without treating the cause. By managing symptoms, patients will usually feel ease or relief. Thus, nursing interventions can be logically inferred and selected, based on the causal related factors and symptoms noted as defining characteristics.

However, with the current NANDA-I taxonomy, for example, *impaired gas exchange* (00030), there are some diagnoses without proper related factors. With these diagnoses, symptom management become the primary nursing intervention.

Problem-focused nursing diagnosis: evaluation reasoning

The last is the *evaluation reasoning component* (▶ **Fig. 3-5**). Evaluation in this model reflects ongoing surveillance and observation; in other words, assessment. The rectangular shape representing surveillance and observation is placed between the defining characteristics and the outcomes. What needs to be observed routinely are the four arrows, which are covered by the rectangle.

We continuously assess signs and symptoms, used as the basis of the diagnosis, and determine a patient's progress toward identified outcomes based on that assessment. We also assess causal related factors and determine how well the patient is resolving the underlying cause, as identified in the selected outcomes.

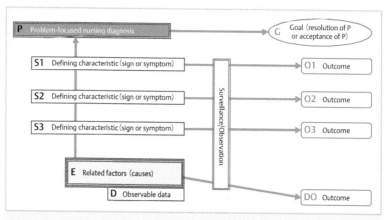

Fig. 3-5 Problem-focused nursing diagnosis: evaluation reasoning

Through surveillance and observation, we evaluate the effectiveness of nursing interventions. Moreover, we evaluate the improvement of the patient's general response (the nursing diagnosis) by evaluating progress toward the identified goal. In addition to those symptoms and signs related to the diagnosis, it is always important to evaluate the general condition of the patient, to ensure patient safety.

Problem-focused nursing diagnosis: integration

So far, we have explained the model by breaking it down into its four components of clinical reasoning. Let's integrate them by reviewing a patient situation (▶ **Fig. 3-6**).

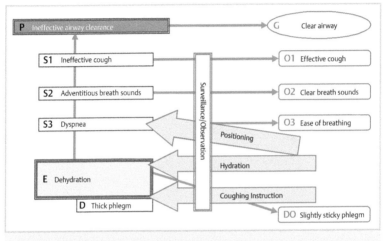

Fig. 3-6 Problem-focused nursing diagnosis: integration

In this case, we have a patient who is exhibiting signs and symptoms of *ineffective airway clearance* (00031), including *ineffective cough, adventitious breath sounds*, and *dyspnea*. The causal related factor is *dehydration*, and it is observed as *thick phlegm*. Although dehydration is not listed in current NANDA-I related factors, it obviously causes this problem. The established goal seeks to resolve the problem, that is *clear airway*. Outcomes linked to the signs and symptoms include *effective cough, clear breath sounds*, and *ease of breathing*. Definitive nursing interventions to remove the cause are *hydration* and *coughing instruction*. We also have symptom management, *positioning*, to relieve the distress caused by *dyspnea*. We continue to assess signs and symptoms, and manifestations of causal factors, to evaluate the effectiveness of nursing interventions. With this patient, what we need to assess includes: his/her *cough, breath sounds, sensation of dyspnea*, and *characteristic of the phlegm*. While assessing these aspects, we can determine the overall condition of the patient, *whether he/she has a clear airway*.

Here, we have three defining characteristics and one related factor to explain the model as simply as possible. If you had identified two defining characteristics, you would also identify two outcomes. If you had identified multiple related factors, you would need to consider multiple definitive interventions as well as multiple outcomes. Please note that it is NOT our intention to suggest that all nursing diagnoses require three defining characteristics and one related factor; that is a simple model for explanatory purposes only.

Clinical Reasoning Model II: Risk Nursing Diagnosis

Now let's examine the clinical reasoning model for risk nursing diagnoses (▶**Fig. 3-7**). As with the model for problem-focused nursing diagnosis, we divide the model into four components.

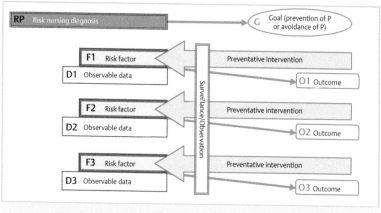

Fig. 3-7 Clinical reasoning model II : risk nursing diagnosis

Risk nursing diagnosis: diagnostic reasoning

▶**Figure 3-8** shows the *diagnostic reasoning* component. The risk nursing diagnosis consists of the following:
- RP: risk for problem (diagnosis label)
- F: risk factors
- D: if a risk factor term is too abstract, it may be helpful to clarify using actual observable data

To identify a risk nursing diagnosis accurately, it is important to perform a thorough nursing assessment and identify *risk factors*. Risk factors are environmental factors, and/or physiological, psychological, genetic, or chemical elements that increase a patient's susceptibility to a response; that is, they basically become those things which cause a problem-focused response. In other words, risk factors become related factors when a patient's response moves from being a risk nursing diagnosis to a problem-focused nursing diagnosis.

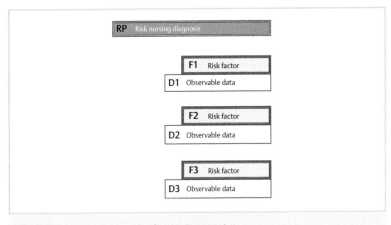

Fig. 3-8 Risk nursing diagnosis: diagnostic reasoning

For instance, *imbalance between oxygen supply/demand* is one of the risk factors of *risk for activity intolerance* (00094). Since we are not able to observe this factor directly, we need to confirm it with observable data, such as *oxygen saturation 92%*, or *patient's report of difficulty breathing during activity*. Risk factors need either to be modifiable or are able to be eliminated with independent nursing interventions.

Risk nursing diagnosis: goal and outcome reasoning

The second part is the *goal and outcome reasoning* component (▸ **Fig. 3-9**). The goal (G) is at the top, and it is always the prevention or avoidance of the problem. Outcomes are generally the resolution or modification of risk factors, and can be logically derived from each risk factor identified.

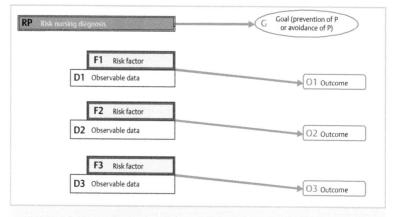

Fig. 3-9 Risk nursing diagnosis: goal and outcome reasoning

Risk nursing diagnosis: nursing intervention reasoning

Next is the nursing intervention reasoning component (▶ **Fig. 3-10**). The three arrows pointing toward the risk factors represent preventative nursing interventions. Preventative nursing interventions are those actions that can remove or modify risk factors, in order to prevent a problem from occurring. Thus, nursing interventions for risk nursing diagnosis can be inferred and selected based on the risk factors identified.

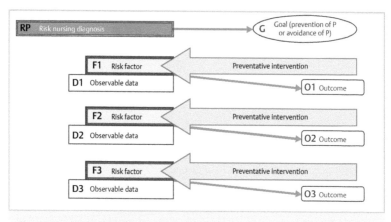

Fig. 3-10 Risk nursing diagnosis: intervention reasoning

Risk nursing diagnosis: evaluation reasoning

The last part of the model is the *evaluation reasoning* component (▶ **Fig. 3-11**). Evaluation in this model requires ongoing surveillance and observations, which again means assessment. Evaluation determines the effectiveness of the preventative nursing interventions that have been implemented. It is also important to evaluate any changes in the condition of the patient.

The rectangular shape representing surveillance and observation is placed between the risk factors and the outcomes. What needs to be observed routinely are represented by the three arrows that are covered by the rectangle. We need to assess those risk factors used as the basis of the diagnosis, and determine the patient's progress toward resolving those risk factors, as identified by the outcomes.

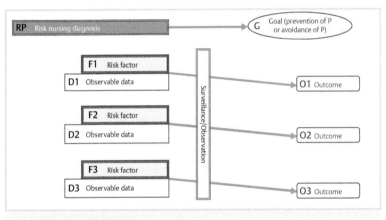

Fig. 3-11 Risk nursing diagnosis: evaluation reasoning

Risk nursing diagnosis: integration

We have explained the model for risk nursing diagnosis by breaking it down into its four components of clinical reasoning. Let's integrate them by reviewing a case (▶ **Fig. 3-12**).

In this case, we have a caregiver who has three risk factors of *risk for caregiver role strain* (00062), including observations of: *caregiver isolation,* as there is *no one with whom she can talk*; *ineffective caregiver coping pattern,* as she has *no effective way to release stress*; and *insufficient respite for caregiver,* because there is *no backup member living nearby.* Based on the diagnosis label, we identify a goal: *caregiver is free from role strain.* In addition, based on the risk factors we can also identify outcomes: *caregiver is not isolated*, *effective caregiver coping pattern*, and *sufficient respite for caregiver*. Preventative interventions to modify risk factors include: *build support system*, *enhance coping skills*, and *provide respite services*. We continue to evaluate the improvement of risk factors to determine the effectiveness of our interventions. What we need to assess includes: *whether or not caregiver is isolated*, *whether stress is released effectively*, and *whether caregiver uses respite when needed*. While assessing these aspects, we determine the overall condition of the caregiver, *whether the caregiver is free from role strain*.

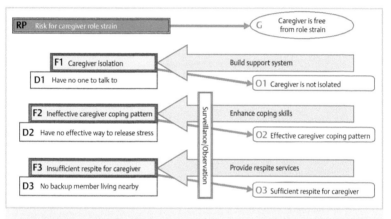

Fig. 3-12 Risk nursing diagnosis: integration

Clinical Reasoning Model III: Health Promotion Nursing Diagnosis

Finally, we will examine the model for health promotion nursing diagnoses (▶**Fig. 3-13**). Here again, we divide the model into four components.

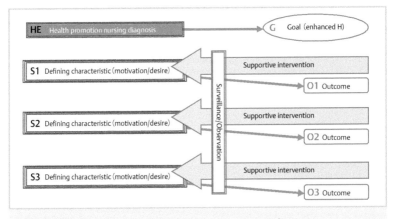

Fig. 3-13 Clinical reasoning model: health promotion nursing diagnosis

Health promotion nursing diagnosis: diagnostic reasoning

▶ **Figure 3-14** shows the *diagnostic reasoning* component. A health promotion nursing diagnosis requires:

- HE: health enhancement, (the diagnosis label)
- S: motivation/desire, (defining characteristics)

The health promotion nursing diagnosis is identified based on the expression of the patient concerning motivation and desire to increase well-being and to actualize health potential. Therefore, defining characteristics represent such statements from the patient. To identify a health promotion nursing diagnosis accurately, it is important to perform a thorough nursing assessment and recognize such statements from the patient. If the patient is unable to express his/her desire, the nurse may determine the condition on the patient's behalf.

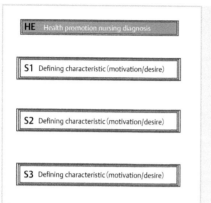

Fig. 3-14 Health promotion nursing diagnosis: diagnostic reasoning

Health promotion nursing diagnosis: goal and outcome reasoning

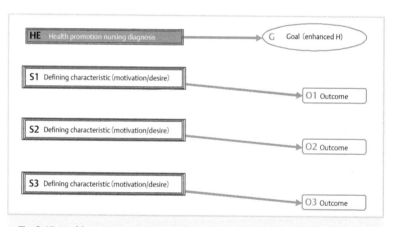

Fig. 3-15 Health promotion nursing diagnosis: goal and outcome reasoning

The second part is the *goal and outcome reasoning* component (▶ **Fig. 3-15**). The final goal (G) is at the top, and it generally represents an enhancement of the focus of the diagnosis. Outcomes are commonly the realization of whatever health behavior the patient desires. Each outcome is logically derived from each defining characteristic.

Health promotion nursing diagnosis: nursing intervention reasoning

Next is the *nursing intervention reasoning* component (▶ **Fig. 3-16**). The three arrows that point toward the defining characteristics represent supportive nursing

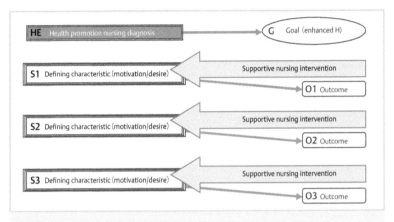

Fig. 3-16 Health promotion nursing diagnosis: nursing intervention reasoning

interventions. Supportive nursing interventions mean those actions that assist the patient in his/her progress toward the identified outcome, while maximizing his/her motivation and desire. Thus, nursing interventions for the diagnosis are inferred and selected based on the confirmed defining characteristics.

Health promotion nursing diagnosis: evaluation reasoning

The last part of the model is the *evaluation reasoning component* (▶ **Fig. 3-17**). Evaluation in this model is based on ongoing surveillance and observation; in other words, assessment. Evaluation determines the effectiveness of the supportive nursing interventions that have been implemented.

The rectangular shape representing surveillance and observation is placed between defining characteristics and the outcomes. What needs to be observed routinely are those three arrows that are covered by the rectangle. We need to assess those defining characteristics used as the basis of the diagnosis, and determine the patient's progress toward outcomes: the realization of the health behavior that the patient desires.

As we explained in Chapter 2, sometimes the patient verbalizes motivation and desire, but makes no progress toward his/her goal. In such a case, it is necessary to discontinue the health promotion nursing diagnosis and consider changing the diagnosis to a risk or problem-focused nursing diagnosis.

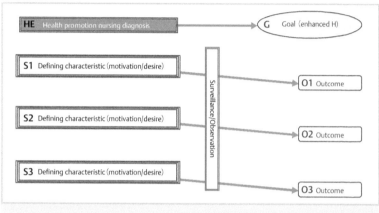

Fig. 3-17 Health promotion nursing diagnosis: evaluation reasoning

Health promotion nursing diagnosis: integration

We explained the model for health promotion nursing diagnosis by breaking it down into its four components of clinical reasoning. Let's integrate these components by reviewing a patient situation (▶**Fig. 3-18**).

Our case is a new employee who is under various stresses at the workplace. He comes to see the employee health nurse and reports that he is not feeling well. At first, the nurse considers the problem-focused nursing diagnosis of *ineffective coping* (00069), but he expresses a desire to enhance *management of stressors, social support,* and *use of emotion-oriented strategies.* Since he is clearly expressing these desire, the nurse identifies the health promotion nursing diagnosis, *readiness for enhanced coping* (00158). The nurse identifies the goal, *enhanced coping,* from the label of the diagnosis. Outcomes identified by linking defining characteristics of the diagnosis include: *enhanced stressor management, enhanced social support,* and *enhanced use of emotion-oriented strategies.* Supportive nursing interventions are aimed at the defining characteristics, which include: *assist with stressor management; provide information regarding social support;* and *assist with the use of emotion-oriented strategies.* The nurse continues to evaluate the realization of the health behavior that he desires, which includes: *management of stressors, social support,* and *use of emotion-oriented strategies.* While assessing these aspects, the nurse determines the overall coping of this employee, or *whether his coping is enhanced.*

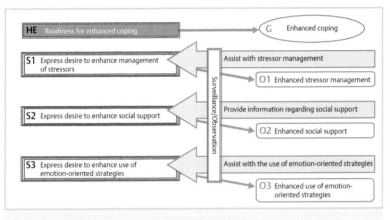

Fig. 3-18 Health promotion nursing diagnosis: integration

4 Quick Understanding of 17 New Nursing Diagnoses

Seventeen new diagnoses were approved by the NANDA-I membership (Herdman & Kamitsuru, 2018, pp. 7–9, ▸**Table 3.1**). On the pages that follow, we provide model cases, key goals and outcomes, and general interventions for these diagnoses to support their use in education, research, and practice. Because these are new nursing diagnoses, work is now needed to identify evidence-based outcomes and interventions. Therefore, in this book we are only providing general guidelines with regard to outcomes and interventions.

Please see the *NANDA International Nursing Diagnoses: Definitions and Classification, 2018–2020* textbook for diagnostic indicators (defining characteristics, related factors, risk factors) and submitters. All references that were used with the submission of these diagnoses are available from the website. www.MediaCenter.Thieme.com

Domain 1. Health Promotion   Class 1. Health Awareness
00262

Readiness for Enhanced Health Literacy

☞ *NANDA International Nursing Diagnoses: Definitions and Classification, 2018–2020,* p. 143

Definition

A pattern of using and developing a set of skills and competencies (literacy, knowledge, motivation, culture, and language) to find, comprehend, evaluate and use health information and concepts to make daily health decisions to promote and maintain health, decrease health risks, and improve overall quality of life, which can be strengthened.

Model case

Mrs. S.A., 48 years old, a preschool teacher, has been experiencing fatigue, hot flashes, and bloating for several months. She wakes up many times during the night, and also has trouble concentrating while reading. She has not had a menstrual period for the last 2 months. She visited a women's clinic and had blood tests to determine the levels of her hormones. The doctor told her that her current symptoms were likely to related to menopause, and explained hormone replacement therapy (HRT) and its possible side effects, such as an increased risk of breast cancer, heart disease, and stroke. This information made her anxious. She needed some time before making her decision, so she left the clinic that day. After returning home, she did an Internet search to learn more about menopause and HRT, and found a local nurse providing menopause counseling. She contacted the nurse and expressed her desire to obtain more information on menopause and HRT, so that she could better understand and make decisions regarding her health care. A few days later, she went to see the nurse to learn more about treatment options for menopause.

Mrs. S.A.'s nursing diagnosis, key goals and outcomes, and general interventions

Nursing diagnosis	Readiness for enhanced health literacy
Defining characteristics	• Expresses desire to enhance personal healthcare decision-making • Expresses desire to enhance understanding of health information to make healthcare choices • Expresses desire to obtain sufficient information to navigate the healthcare system
Ultimate goal	Enhanced health literacy
Key outcomes	• Enhanced personal healthcare decision-making • Enhanced understanding of health information to make healthcare choices • Sufficient information to navigate the healthcare system
General interventions	• Support in making healthcare decisions • Assist to understand health information • Assist to obtain information

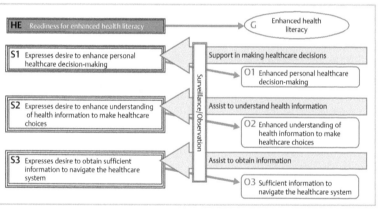

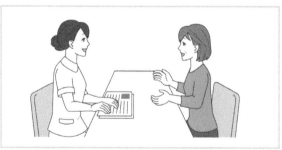

Domain 2. Nutrition   Class 1. Ingestion
00269

Ineffective Adolescent Eating Dynamics

☞ *NANDA International Nursing Diagnoses: Definitions and Classification, 2018–2020,* p. 163

Definition

Altered attitudes and behaviors resulting in over or under eating patterns that compromise nutritional health.

Model case

Ms. A.T., 16 years old, is a sophomore in high school. She is under a lot of pressure to get excellent grades in school and states she has excessive stress and anxiety related to this. She gained 44 pounds (20 kg) in the past year, and has begun to experience low self-esteem, which she believes is due to bullying at school and on social media. She mentions that other students make fun of her, call her names, and constantly laugh at her weight. She tells the nurse that she is always hungry, frequently snacks, eats foods from fast food restaurants, and frequently buys snacks. Her parents have started to make negative comments about her weight, and have started measuring all of her food at mealtimes at home. They will not allow her to eat anything more than what they give her during meals when she is at home. She dislikes eating at home now because she finds mealtimes very uncomfortable. She says the only thing that makes her feel better is when she eats.

Ms. A.T.'s nursing diagnosis, key goals and outcomes, and general interventions

Nursing diagnosis	Ineffective adolescent eating dynamics
Related factors	▪ Excessive stress ▪ Changes to self-esteem upon entering puberty ▪ Excessive family mealtime control
Defining characteristics	▪ Complains of hunger between meals ▪ Frequent snacking ▪ Overeating ▪ Frequently eating from fast food restaurants
Ultimate goal	Effective adolescent eating dynamics

(Continued)

(Continued)

Key outcomes
- Satisfy with meals and small serving nutritious food throughout the day
- Improved quality of food being consumed
- Normal stress levels
- Improved self-esteem
- Parents provide supportive eating environment

General interventions
- Empower to develop nutritious, good tasting meal plan
- Encourage healthy snacks to supplement meals throughout the day
- Empower to develop activity plan to manage stress and support weight loss
- Educate parents about need to provide supportive eating environment
- Identify support group for adolescents with low self-esteem

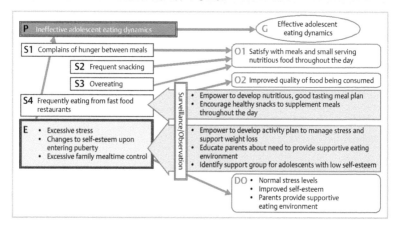

P Ineffective adolescent eating dynamics

G Effective adolescent eating dynamics

S1 Complains of hunger between meals

S2 Frequent snacking

S3 Overeating

S4 Frequently eating from fast food restaurants

E
- Excessive stress
- Changes to self-esteem upon entering puberty
- Excessive family mealtime control

Surveillance/Observation

O1 Satisfy with meals and small serving nutritious food throughout the day

O2 Improved quality of food being consumed

- Empower to develop nutritious, good tasting meal plan
- Encourage healthy snacks to supplement meals throughout the day

- Empower to develop activity plan to manage stress and support weight loss
- Educate parents about need to provide supportive eating environment
- Identify support group for adolescents with low self-esteem

DO
- Normal stress levels
- Improved self-esteem
- Parents provide supportive eating environment

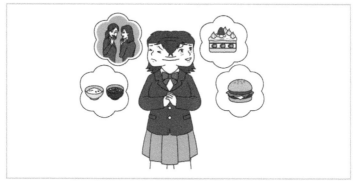

Domain 2. Nutrition   Class 1. Ingestion
00270

Ineffective Child Eating Dynamics

☞ *NANDA International Nursing Diagnoses: Definitions and Classification, 2018–2020,* p. 164

Definition

Altered attitudes, behaviors and influences on child eating patterns resulting in compromised nutritional health.

Model case

H.W. is an 8-year-old boy. He has an older brother who no longer lives at home. His brother is obese and had significant struggles in school with forming friendships and participating in events. His parents blame themselves for allowing their first son to become obese, because they never forbid him anything he desired. They are determined not to allow him to suffer the same social difficulties as his brother. They have put a lock on the door to the pantry, and he is not allowed to have any food other than at meal times. His school lunches are prepared by his mother and consist of a small amount of vegetables and fruits. He is not allowed to carry any money with him, so he cannot purchase any foods outside the home. During meals at home, he is allowed only one cup of vegetables, 2 ounces of tofu or meat, and a piece of fruit. He is not allowed to have rice, breads, noodles, or deserts. His mother weighs every portion. If he asks for his desired food choices, his father becomes very upset and yells at him. He is told that he is too young to know what foods are good for him, and that his parents will decide when, what, and how much he eats. During the meals, his parents lecture him constantly about how important it is that he stay thin so that he will have an easier life than his brother. If he tells his parents he is still hungry, he is asked if he wants to end up like his brother, and is sent to his room to consider the consequences of overeating.

Boy H.W.'s nursing diagnosis, key goals and outcomes, and general interventions

Nursing diagnosis	Ineffective child eating dynamics
Related factors	• Excessive parental control over child's eating experience • Stressful mealtimes • Inability to divide eating responsibility between parent and child
Defining characteristics	• Complains of hunger between meals • Undereating
Ultimate goal	Effective child eating dynamics
Key outcomes	• Satisfy with meals and small serving nutritious food throughout the day • Appropriate nutritional intake for child's healthy growth and development • Reasonable parental control over child's eating experience • Stress-free mealtimes • Demonstrates ability to divide eating responsibility between parent and child
General interventions	• Discuss with parents about appropriate parental control over child's eating experience • Assist parents in understanding the importance of a pleasant, stress-free meal time • Work with parents to divide eating responsibility between themselves and their child

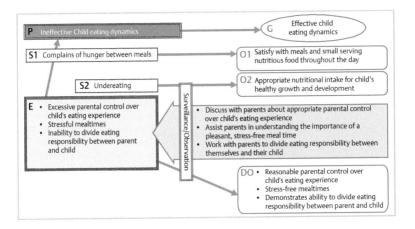

P Ineffective Child eating dynamics

G Effective child eating dynamics

S1 Complains of hunger between meals

O1 Satisfy with meals and small serving nutritious food throughout the day

S2 Undereating

O2 Appropriate nutritional intake for child's healthy growth and development

E
- Excessive parental control over child's eating experience
- Stressful mealtimes
- Inability to divide eating responsibility between parent and child

Surveillance/Observation

- Discuss with parents about appropriate parental control over child's eating experience
- Assist parents in understanding the importance of a pleasant, stress-free meal time
- Work with parents to divide eating responsibility between themselves and their child

DO
- Reasonable parental control over child's eating experience
- Stress-free mealtimes
- Demonstrates ability to divide eating responsibility between parent and child

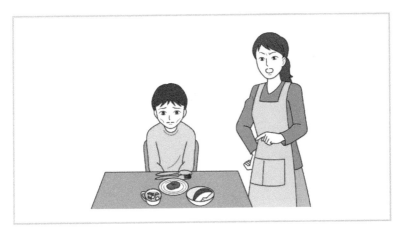

Domain 2. Nutrition   Class 1. Ingestion
00271

Ineffective Infant Feeding Dynamics

☞ *NANDA International Nursing Diagnoses: Definitions and Classification, 2018–2020,* p. 166

Definition

Altered parental feeding behaviors resulting in over or under eating patterns.

Model case

Mr. and Mrs. Y have a 3-year-old son and a baby girl, M.Y. aged 2 months. They have also been raising Mrs. Y's 16-year-old sister E.F. and 14-year-old brother, D.F., for the past three years, after their parents died in an automobile accident. Both siblings were badly hurt in the accident; there has also been a lot of psychological trauma. At a scheduled well baby visit, the nurse notices that M.Y. seems to be gaining weight very fast. She asks Mrs. Y how she feeds her baby. Mrs. Y explains that she and her husband both work two different jobs to support the family. Her children are often cared for by an older neighbor woman, or by Mrs. Y's siblings. Her sister E.F. in particular has formed a strong bond with M.Y., and cares for her frequently when she is not in school. E.F. tells the nurse that it makes her very sad when M.Y. fusses or cries, and so she immediately offers her a bottle. She tries to make M.Y. finish the bottle, even if she seems disinterested, because she believes this will calm the infant. In the past week, E.F. began providing rice porridge to M.Y. when she became fussy, because she saw this on the internet as an appropriate food for babies. She feels that the rice stops M.Y. from crying, and that is her top priority. This was a big surprise to Mrs. Y, who was unaware that E.F. had introduced solid food. In contrast, E.F. criticizes the neighbor, because she will allow M.Y. to fuss and does not feed her unless she cannot console her in other ways. E.F. feels this is cruel. Mrs. Y, tells the nurse that she tries to breastfeed when she is home, and provides breastmilk for her bottle feedings, but M.Y. seems to have more trouble with breastfeeding than bottle feeding, which she finds very frustrating as her mother.

Baby M.'s nursing diagnosis, key goals and outcomes, and general interventions

Nursing diagnosis	Ineffective infant feeding dynamics
Related factors	• Lack of knowledge of appropriate methods of feeding infant for each stage of development • Multiple caregivers
Defining characteristics	• Inappropriate transition to solid foods • Overeating
Ultimate goal	Effective infant feeding dynamics
Key outcomes	• Appropriate food types and amount for infant's stage of development • All caregivers understand appropriate methods of feeding infant for each stage of development • All caregivers understand their responsibilities for feeding infant
General interventions	• Assist all caregivers to understand appropriate methods of feeding infant for each stage of development • Assist all caregivers to understand their responsibility in feeding infant

Quick Understanding of 17 New Nursing Diagnoses

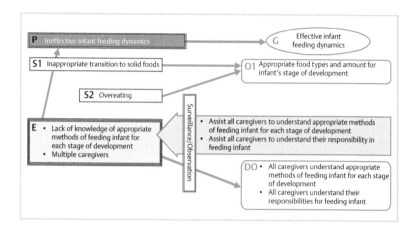

P Ineffective infant feeding dynamics

G Effective infant feeding dynamics

S1 Inappropriate transition to solid foods

O1 Appropriate food types and amount for infant's stage of development

S2 Overeating

Surveillance/Observation

E
- Lack of knowledge of appropriate methods of feeding infant for each stage of development
- Multiple caregivers

- Assist all caregivers to understand appropriate methods of feeding infant for each stage of development
- Assist all caregivers to understand their responsibility in feeding infant

DO
- All caregivers understand appropriate methods of feeding infant for each stage of development
- All caregivers understand their responsibilities for feeding infant

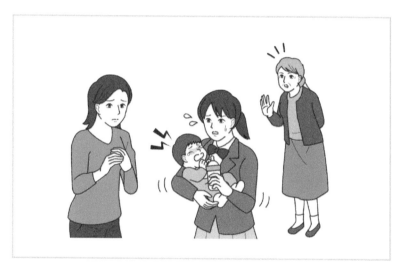

Domain 2. Nutrition   Class 4. Metabolism
00263

Risk for Metabolic Imbalance Syndrome

☞ *NANDA International Nursing Diagnoses: Definitions and Classification, 2018–2020,* p. 181

Definition

Susceptible to a toxic cluster of biochemical and physiological factors associated with the development of cardiovascular disease arising from obesity and type 2 diabetes, which may compromise health.

Model case

Mr. J.O., is a 56-year-old man, working as a sales manager for a publishing company. He visits his local clinic with the urging of his wife, because he has not seen a health care provider in more than 10 years. He indicates he does not have time for appointments, and is generally healthy. His only complaint is "constant fatigue," which he attributes to his work. He travels 3–5 days/week for work, and often works 14–16 hours/day. His work role is very high stress, and the environment is a competitive one; he rarely takes a day off for relaxation. He fears that if he is not working, someone younger will try to take his place. He is about 50 pounds (23 kg) above his ideal body weight, and the nurse tells him he is very close to being considered obese. When she asks about his nutrition, he says that, because of his work life, he eats out every day, often for all of his meals. He tries to sleep "every minute he can," so he doesn't have time to eat breakfast at home. He buys something to eat at the train station when he arrives at his work stop, and goes to the local convenience store for lunch and some snacks. When he is not traveling, he usually orders take out or fast food delivery for dinner, which he eats in the office as he is working on paperwork. When he is traveling, he often has business dinners with clients, so he is likely to have several alcoholic drinks as well as large dinners. He notes that he "doesn't have time" for any exercise, so his only activity is the walking he does to and from the train, which is about a five minute walk. He primarily sits at his computer screen when in the office, or at the meeting with potential clients. His blood work includes: plasma insulin at the 70th percentile, fasting blood sugar is 112 mg/dL, total glucose is 145 mg/dL, HDL 39 mg/dL. Additionally, his waist circumference is 98 cm/38.5 inches, and his blood pressure is 134/88.

Mr. J.O.'s nursing diagnosis, key goals and outcomes, and general interventions

Nursing diagnosis	Risk for metabolic imbalance syndrome
Risk factors	• Overweight (00233) • Sedentary lifestyle (00168) • Stress overload (00177)
Ultimate goal	Avoidance of metabolic imbalance syndrome
Key outcomes	• Decrease body weight by 8–10 pounds in the next six months. • Participate in a minimum of 30 minutes of moderate activity per day • Develop coping mechanisms to decrease stress levels
General interventions	• Support to adopt a healthier nutritional pattern, including selection of more healthy options at restaurants • Discuss meals he can prepare and take to work for at least one meal/day • Assist to adapt his work requirements to support activity (e.g., standing desk, taking 5-minute walk breaks every 45 minutes) • Encourage use of mindful meditation, guided imagery to help with stress levels

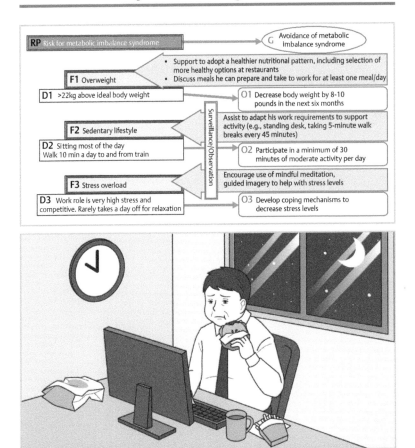

▶ **Authors' note** ◀

Metabolic syndrome is a well-known medical diagnosis found in ICD-10, and it is defined as "a cluster of metabolic risk factors for cardiovascular diseases and type 2 diabetes mellitus." Therefore, *metabolic syndrome* appears to represent the same health condition that this particular new NANDA-I risk nursing diagnosis is intended to capture. Since this diagnosis represents increased susceptibility to clusters of risk factors, it is difficult to differentiate this from *metabolic syndrome.* Moreover, all references used by the authors of this diagnosis are related to metabolic syndrome, which increases the confusion. Finally, all risk factors of this diagnosis are nursing diagnoses, which is not a NANDA-I requirement. We would like to encourage further validation of this diagnosis.

Domain 4. Activity/rest   Class 3. Energy balance
00273

Imbalanced Energy Field

☞ *NANDA International Nursing Diagnoses: Definitions and Classification, 2018–2020,* p. 225

Definition

A disruption in the vital flow of human energy that is normally a continuous whole and is unique, dynamic, creative, and nonlinear.

Model case

Ms. A.C., 38 years old, is a self-employed tax accountant. She has recently divorced after a long international custody battle. She has been raising two girls, 7 and 10 years old, with help from her mother and sister who live nearby. Her father was recently hospitalized due to a severe stroke. She is not getting as much help from her family as she had hoped to receive. She has sleep problems, headaches, and a loss of appetite. She lost nearly 7 kg (15.4 pound) in the past few months. She went to see her family doctor, but he did not find anything wrong. A friend of hers recommended a nurse who practiced holistic nursing, so she visited the clinic. She told the nurse that she has been very stressed from these things that have happened to her recently. During the energy assessments, the nurse found arrhythmic energy field patterns, and congested energy flow.

Miss A.C.'s nursing diagnosis, key goals and outcomes, and general interventions

Nursing diagnosis	Imbalanced energy field
Related factors	• Anxiety • Excessive stress
Defining characteristics	▪ Arrhythmic energy field patterns ▪ Congestion of the energy flow
Ultimate goal	Balanced energy field
Key outcomes	▪ Rhythmic energy field patterns ▪ Uncongested energy flow ▪ Reduced anxiety ▪ Reduced stress level
General interventions	▪ Therapeutic touch ▪ Assist to identify effective stress reduction method ▪ Encourage use of meditation

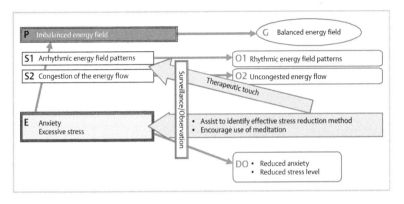

P	Imbalanced energy field		**G**	Balanced energy field
S1	Arrhythmic energy field patterns		**O1**	Rhythmic energy field patterns
S2	Congestion of the energy flow		**O2**	Uncongested energy flow

Surveillance/Observation

Therapeutic touch

E	Anxiety Excessive stress

- Assist to identify effective stress reduction method
- Encourage use of meditation

DO • Reduced anxiety
• Reduced stress level

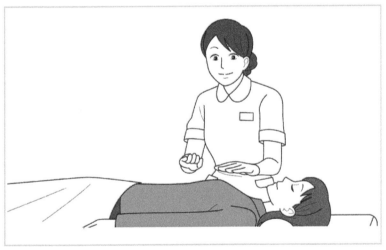

Risk for Unstable Blood Pressure

☞ *NANDA International Nursing Diagnoses: Definitions and Classification, 2018–2020,* p. 235

Definition

Susceptible to fluctuating forces of blood flowing through arterial vessels, which may compromise health.

Model case

Mr. H.Y., 55 years old, runs a textile factory. Elevated blood pressure (180/110 mmHg) was detected during his yearly health examination at his work site. He drinks 1–2 glasses of beer and smokes one pack of cigarettes daily. He often eats out with his employees, and likes spicy and salty foods. His body mass index (BMI) is 32. At the clinic, he was diagnosed with hypertension, and was prescribed medication. He also received instructions to modify his lifestyle and choose a healthy diet. In the following month, during the clinic visit, he told the nurse that he had been experiencing dizziness during the past week. He noted that this happened mostly when he got out of bed in the morning. He also told her that changing his lifestyle is very difficult, and he often forgets to take his medication because he is very busy. His blood pressure was 165/110 mmHg.

Mr. H.Y.'s nursing diagnosis, key goals and outcomes, and general interventions

Nursing diagnosis	Risk for unstable blood pressure
Risk factors	• Inconsistency with medication regimen • Orthostasis
Ultimate goal	Stable blood pressure
Key outcomes	• Follow medication regimen • Prevent orthostasis
General interventions	• Explain the importance of medication regimen • Work with patient to incorporate regimen into his work schedule • Recommend assistive device to remind patient to take medication (e.g., pill box with alarm reminder) • Help to understand the cause of orthostasis

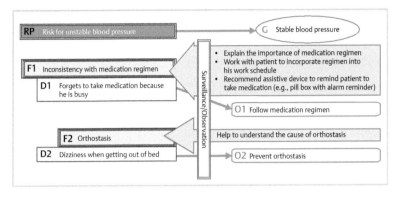

RP Risk for unstable blood pressure	G Stable blood pressure
F1 Inconsistency with medication regimen	• Explain the importance of medication regimen • Work with patient to incorporate regimen into his work schedule • Recommend assistive device to remind patient to take medication (e.g., pill box with alarm reminder)
D1 Forgets to take medication because he is busy	O1 Follow medication regimen
F2 Orthostasis	Help to understand the cause of orthostasis
D2 Dizziness when getting out of bed	O2 Prevent orthostasis

Surveillance/Observation

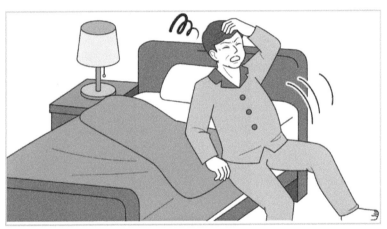

Domain 9. Coping/stress tolerance   Class 1. Post-trauma responses
00260

Risk for Complicated Immigration Transition

☞ *NANDA International Nursing Diagnoses: Definitions and Classification, 2018–2020,* p. 315

Definition

Susceptible to experiencing negative feelings (loneliness, fear, anxiety) in response to unsatisfactory consequences and cultural barriers to one's immigration transition, which may compromise health.

Model case

Mr. J.A.'s family fled from its country of origin 9 months ago, due to the intensifying civil war. He came to the host country with his wife, and their two children, a 9-year-old son and 7-year-old daughter, but they left their sick parents back in their country of origin. He was a high school mathematics teacher in his home country. When the family arrived at the host country, none of them spoke or understood the local language. Although they were eligible to receive housing, financial, and medical assistance during the first year, it took them a few months to learn about such information. They live in a small apartment with another family, but it is too cramped to accommodate two families. His children were able to easily blend in with the local school and culture, and are learning the language very well. They have seemed embarrassed by their parents' inability to adapt to the language and customs of their new country. Soon, however, the family will be cut off from immigrant assistance, so he has been looking for a job. However, he could only find a low-skill job due to the language barriers. He notes he has been feeling depressed.

Mr. J.A.'s nursing diagnosis, key goals and outcomes, and general interventions

Nursing diagnosis	Risk for complicated immigration transition
Risk factors	• Available work below educational preparation • Language barriers in host country • Overcrowded housing • Parent-child conflicts related to enculturation in the host country
Ultimate goal	Smooth immigration transition
Key outcomes	• Increased satisfaction with work • Overcome language barriers • Improved living environment • Enhanced parent-child mutual understanding and cooperation related to enculturation in the host country
General interventions	• Provide assistance to find job training opportunities • Provide assistance to find language classes • Provide assistance to find better housing • Enhance parent-child mutual understanding and cooperation related to enculturation in the host country • Encourage stress relief strategies in which the entire family can participate

Quick Understanding of 17 New Nursing Diagnoses

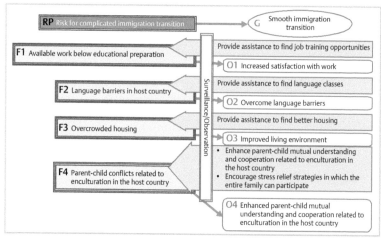

RP Risk for complicated immigration transition → **G** Smooth immigration transition

F1 Available work below educational preparation

Provide assistance to find job training opportunities

O1 Increased satisfaction with work

F2 Language barriers in host country

Provide assistance to find language classes

O2 Overcome language barriers

F3 Overcrowded housing

Provide assistance to find better housing

O3 Improved living environment

F4 Parent-child conflicts related to enculturation in the host country

- Enhance parent-child mutual understanding and cooperation related to enculturation in the host country
- Encourage stress relief strategies in which the entire family can participate

O4 Enhanced parent-child mutual understanding and cooperation related to enculturation in the host country

Surveillance/Observation

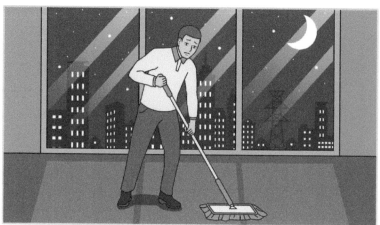

<u>**Domain 9. Coping/stress tolerance   Class 3. Neurobehavioral stress**</u>
00258

Acute Substance Withdrawal Syndrome

☞ *NANDA International Nursing Diagnoses: Definitions and Classification, 2018–2020,* p. 351

Definition

Serious, multifactorial sequelae following abrupt cessation of an addictive compound.

Model case

Mr. K.F., a 60-year-old man, was admitted to the hospital through the emergency department, after a neighbor called for an ambulance when he fell down a flight of stairs in his apartment building. He appears emaciated, and was admitted to the hospital with a blood alcohol level of 0.38, and a fractured humerus and femur that would require surgical intervention. After being hospitalized approximately 60 hours, he began to become acutely confused, very anxious and has begun to develop significant tremors. His blood pressure is 188/112 mmHg, his respirations are 32/minute, and his heart rate is 166 bpm. He is diaphoretic, complains of severe nausea, and has been unable to sleep for more than 22 hours. He is trying to get out of bed constantly, despite his leg being in traction and his arm in a cast, saying he has to "get away from them." He appears to be hallucinating. His daughter is listed as the emergency contact, and when called, she tells the nurse that her father was diagnosed with psychological issues when she was younger, but she does not know the name of the diagnosis. Her mother would never talk about this. She indicates that her father is an alcoholic, and she also says that the family has suspected that he abuses illicit drugs. He left the family home more than two years ago when his wife demanded that he seek treatment, and she does not know where he has been living.

Mr. K.F.'s nursing diagnosis, key goals and outcomes, and general interventions

Nursing diagnosis	Acute substance withdrawal syndrome
Related factors	• Heavy use of an addictive substance over time • Sudden cessation of an addictive substance
Defining characteristics	• Acute confusion (00128) • Anxiety (00146) • Disturbed sleep pattern (00198) • Nausea (00134) • Risk for injury (00035)
Ultimate goal	Safely manage acute substance withdrawal
Key outcomes	• Well-controlled symptoms to reach nonproblematic levels • Improved health and functional status • Free from physical injury
General interventions	• Maintain a quiet, semi-dark, calm environment • Provide simple explanations for care • Consider use of chemical and/or physical restraints to avoid injury, in conjunction with care team

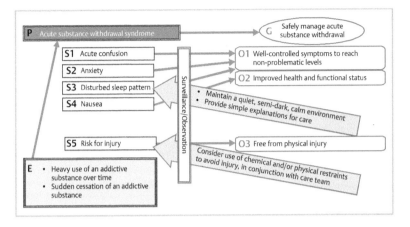

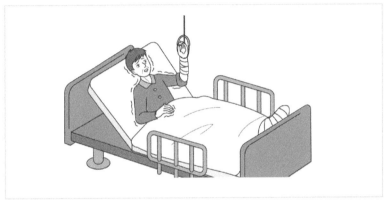

► Authors' note ◄

Unfortunately, patients in many countries struggle with substance abuse and withdrawal states from addictive substances, and nurses provide their care. A withdrawal state is classified in ICD-10, and defined as "a group of symptoms of variable clustering and severity occurring on absolute or relative withdrawal of a substance after repeated, and usually prolonged and/or high-dose, use of that substance." The question we raise is, how is this new diagnosis different from a *withdrawal state*? Moreover, nurses are not able to modify some of the related factors to prevent this syndrome to happen, such as *heavy use of an addictive substance over time*, and *sudden cessation of an addictive substance*. These factors may fit better under at-risk populations. We would like to encourage further validation of this diagnosis.

Domain 9. Coping/stress tolerance   Class 3. Neurobehavioral stress
00259

Risk for Acute Substance Withdrawal Syndrome

☞ *NANDA International Nursing Diagnoses: Definitions and Classification, 2018–2020,* p. 352

Definition

Susceptible to serious, multifactorial sequelae following abrupt cessation of an addictive compound, which may compromise health.

Model case

Miss N.M., a 31-year-old woman, is a binge drinker, often drinking so much alcohol on weekends that she is unable to remember anything that happened. She indicates this behavior started in college and has continued the past few years in her professional career. She also uses marijuana occasionally, and drinks 1–2 glasses of wine after work during the week. She has been brought to the clinic by her boyfriend who is concerned about how much weight she has lost in the past year, and what he says are lapses in her memory. He says that after a conflict between the two of them, she stopped drinking yesterday and he is concerned that she may have problems withdrawing from the substance. She tells the nurse that her boyfriend is exaggerating; she just enjoys relaxing and having a good time on the weekend after a hard week at work. However, she does admit that there have been a few Monday mornings when she has been unable to go to her job, because she is too sick with nausea or headaches. The nurse begins to talk with her about her alcohol use, possible consequences she might face if she is not able to decrease or control her alcohol, and interventions that she could recommend to help her address her overuse of alcohol. Her boyfriend is very supportive of her getting professional help, so she agrees to see an addiction specialist for evaluation and treatment.

Miss N.M.'s nursing diagnosis, key goals and outcomes, and general interventions

Nursing diagnosis	Risk for acute substance withdrawal syndrome
Risk factors	• Heavy use of an addictive substance over time • Malnutrition • Sudden cessation of an addictive substance
Ultimate goal	Prevent acute substance withdrawal syndrome
Key outcomes	• Understand drivers behind the use of substances and develop plan to manage these drivers without substances • Develop plan to find enjoyment other than alcohol • Develop coping mechanisms for dealing with stress • Stable nutritional status
General interventions	• Refer to addiction specialist for assessment and treatment • Work with patient to understand drivers that lead to use of substances • Assist to find enjoyment other than alcohol • Provide help to develop coping mechanisms • Provide encouragement and information to key support person • Support nutritional health through use of foods high in protein, folate, thiamine, or vitamin B12

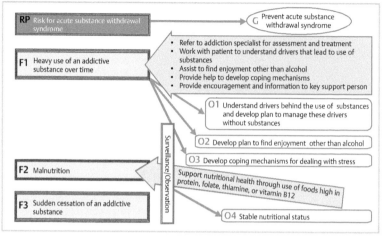

RP Risk for acute substance withdrawal syndrome

G Prevent acute substance withdrawal syndrome

F1 Heavy use of an addictive substance over time

- Refer to addiction specialist for assessment and treatment
- Work with patient to understand drivers that lead to use of substances
- Assist to find enjoyment other than alcohol
- Provide help to develop coping mechanisms
- Provide encouragement and information to key support person

O1 Understand drivers behind the use of substances and develop plan to manage these drivers without substances

O2 Develop plan to find enjoyment other than alcohol

O3 Develop coping mechanisms for dealing with stress

F2 Malnutrition

Surveillance/Observation

Support nutritional health through use of foods high in protein, folate, thiamine, or vitamin B12

F3 Sudden cessation of an addictive substance

O4 Stable nutritional status

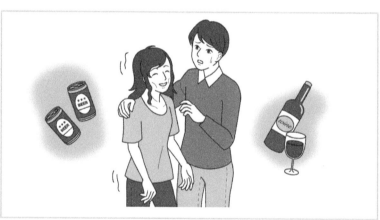

Neonatal Abstinence Syndrome

☞ *NANDA International Nursing Diagnoses: Definitions and Classification, 2018–2020,* p. 358

Definition

A constellation of withdrawal symptoms observed in newborns as a result of in-utero exposure to addicting substances, or as a consequence of postnatal pharmacological pain management.

Model case

Baby boy S is a 31-week gestation infant, born three days ago to a mother using methamphetamines and marijuana during pregnancy. He is in the neonatal intensive care unit with some mild respiratory distress and inability to independently maintain his thermoregulation. Currently, his vital signs indicate tachypnea and moderate hyperthermia. As the nurse observes him, she notices many stress responses, such as finger splaying, impaired motor tone, frequent bradycardic and oxygen desaturation episodes. He has frequent changes in his sleep-wake state, often going from sleep to a startled awake state with crying. He primarily refuses to take nutrition orally, and when he does suck, he is unable to take much formula by mouth without oral cyanosis and desaturations occurring; he is primarily receiving feedings via gavage tube. He also has moderate regurgitation after feeds. He becomes very stressed when he is touched, makes no attempt at eye contact, and displays multiple stress signals during any intervention or attempt to comfort.

Baby boy S.'s nursing diagnosis, key goals and outcomes, and general interventions

Nursing diagnosis	Neonatal abstinence syndrome
Related factors	• To be developed
Defining characteristics	• Disorganized infant behavior (00116)
	• Neurobehavioral stress
	• Disturbed sleep pattern (00198)
	• Risk for ineffective thermoregulation (00274)
	• Ineffective infant feeding pattern (00107)
	• Risk for impaired attachment (00058)
Ultimate goal	Manage and minimize neonate's withdrawal symptoms
Key outcomes	• Organized infant behavior
	• Seizure free
	• Normal sleeping pattern
	• Stable thermoregulation
	• Appropriate weight gain
	• Attachment formation
General interventions	• Implement continuous minimal stimulation practices with dim light and low noise
	• Initiate gentle handling, demand feeding, and careful avoidance of waking the sleeping infant
	• Implement swaddling to lessen stimulation, decrease crying times, and promote sleep that is more sustained
	• Frequent feeds with high-calorie formula to meet nutritional and metabolic demands
	• Work with parents to initiate kangaroo care

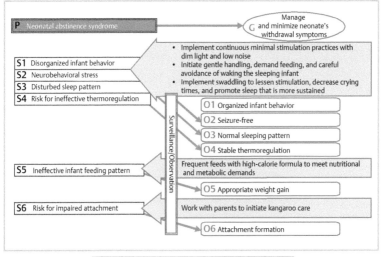

P Neonatal abstinence syndrome	→	Manage ₲ and minimize neonate's withdrawal symptoms

S1 Disorganized infant behavior
S2 Neurobehavioral stress
S3 Disturbed sleep pattern
S4 Risk for ineffective thermoregulation

- Implement continuous minimal stimulation practices with dim light and low noise
- Initiate gentle handling, demand feeding, and careful avoidance of waking the sleeping infant
- Implement swaddling to lessen stimulation, decrease crying times, and promote sleep that is more sustained

O1 Organized infant behavior
O2 Seizure-free
O3 Normal sleeping pattern
O4 Stable thermoregulation

Surveillance/Observation

S5 Ineffective infant feeding pattern

Frequent feeds with high-calorie formula to meet nutritional and metabolic demands

O5 Appropriate weight gain

S6 Risk for impaired attachment

Work with parents to initiate kangaroo care

O6 Attachment formation

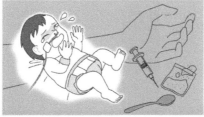

► Authors' note ◄

This diagnosis was approved before NANDA-I introduced two new categories to the terminology, *at-risk populations* and *associated conditions.* Two of the original related factors were subsequently categorized as *at-risk populations.* Therefore, modifiable related factors common to a specific cluster of nursing diagnoses need to be developed for this diagnosis. Logically thinking, a common etiological factor of the identified nursing diagnoses is withdrawal of an addictive substance from the neonate. However, nurses are not able to modify that etiology, because the substance has already been withdrawn from this infant when the nurse encounters him/her for the first time in the NICU. We would therefore argue that nurses need to focus on symptom control, and so we must consider whether or not the identified nursing diagnoses within the defining characteristics list are symptoms. As previously noted, a withdrawal state is classified in ICD-10, and defined as "a group of symptoms of variable clustering and severity occurring on absolute or relative withdrawal of a substance after repeated, and usually prolonged and/or high-dose, use of that substance." Therefore, another question we raise is, how is this new diagnosis different from a *withdrawal state*? We would like to encourage further validation of this diagnosis.

Domain 11. Safety/protection   Class 1. Infection
00266

Risk for Surgical Site Infection

☞ *NANDA International Nursing Diagnoses: Definitions and Classification, 2018–2020,* p. 383

Definition

Susceptible to invasion of pathogenic organisms at surgical site, which may compromise health.

Model case

Mr. Y.S., 75 years old, is a retired realtor. For the last 5 years, he sometimes experienced discomfort and pain in both knees; however, he decided to try to ignore it, and did not seek treatment. Recently, he has begun to experience significant pain when he walks or moves the joint. He went to see an orthopedic specialist, and he was diagnosed with advanced osteoarthritis of the knee. The doctor told him that he needs knee replacement surgery. In addition, the surgeon told him that both knees should be replaced at one time, to lower complications. He is taking medications for diabetes mellitus and hypertension, and is being treated for obesity (BMI 34). He smokes one pack of cigarettes daily. The doctor advised him to lose weight and modify his lifestyle immediately to prepare for the surgery scheduled 6 months later.

Mr. Y.S.'s nursing diagnosis, key goals and outcomes, and general interventions

Nursing diagnosis	Risk for surgical site infection
Risk factors	• Obesity • Smoking
Ultimate goal	No surgical site infection
Key outcomes	▪ Weight reduction ▪ Weight management behaviors ▪ Smoking cessation
General interventions	▪ Provide nutrition counseling ▪ Develop plan to increase activity/exercise that doesn't impact his knees ▪ Assist to identify effective method for smoking cessation

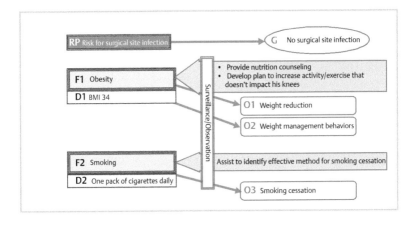

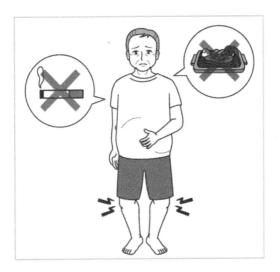

▶ Authors' note ◀

This diagnosis was approved before NANDA-I introduced two new categories to the terminology, *at-risk populations* and *associated conditions*. Most of the suggested original risk factors are now found under these two categories. The current risk factors are not something that nurses can treat if a surgery is imminent, because they all require time. We would like to encourage further development of this diagnosis.

Domain 11. Safety/protection   Class 2. Physical injury
00261

Risk for Dry Mouth

☞ *NANDA International Nursing Diagnoses: Definitions and Classification, 2018–2020,* p. 389

Definition

Susceptible to discomfort or damage to the oral mucosa due to reduced quantity or quality of saliva to moisten the mucosa, which may compromise health.

Model case

Mr. S.T., 75 years old, has a history of chronic obstructive pulmonary disease (COPD). One night, he was brought to the emergency department (ED) by an ambulance with complaints of severe dyspnea. His SpO2 was 88%, and his blood gas results were: pH 7.30, PaO2 55, and PaCO2 70 mmHg. On arrival, he was alert and oriented, appeared very excited/anxious, but gradually developed lethargy. The ED physician diagnosed him with an acute exacerbation of COPD, and ordered the use of non invasive positive pressure ventilation via face mask. His SpO2 improved to 90%, and he was transferred to the pulmonary unit. During his admission to the unit, his wife told the nurse that he did not drink or eat anything most of the day because of his condition. After a short time on the unit, he became agitated and complained of discomfort and pain from the mask. A small dose of analgesic was administered, and before long, he calmed down and began to rest with the mask in place.

Mr. S.T.'s nursing diagnosis, key goals and outcomes, and general interventions

Nursing diagnosis	Risk for dry mouth
Risk factors	• Dehydration • Excessive stress • Excitement
Ultimate goal	Maintain moist mouth
Key outcomes	• Adequate hydration • Reduced stress level • Reduced agitation
General interventions	• Provide fluid if appropriate • Reduce environmental and situational stressors • Provide soothing environment • Apply mouth moisturizer

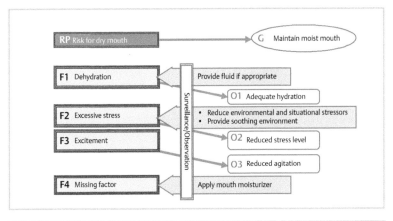

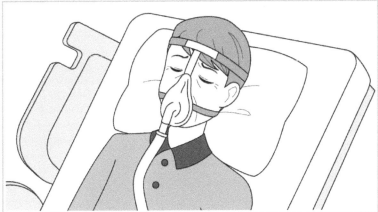

▶ Authors' note ◀

Mouth moisturizing gel or spray is generally used for patients with this risk, and for those who already have the problem. When we reviewed the basis of the nursing intervention, *apply mouth moisturizer,* with the clinical reasoning model, there is no corresponding risk factor. It is possible that the phenomena of this diagnosis can be expanded with a problem-focused diagnosis. We would like to encourage further validation of this diagnosis.

<u>**Domain 11. Safety/protection   Class 2. Physical injury**</u>
00268

Risk for Venous Thromboembolism

☞ *NANDA International Nursing Diagnoses: Definitions and Classification, 2018–2020,* p. 414

Definition

Susceptible to the development of a blood clot in a deep vein, commonly in the thigh, calf or upper extremity, which can break off and lodge in another vessel, which may compromise health.

Model case

Mrs. E.K., 65 years old, is diagnosed with cervical cancer, and had a total abdominal hysterectomy this morning. She has a history of right breast cancer and had a right breast lumpectomy ten years ago. After the previous surgery, she developed a thromboembolism. She also has a history of a cerebral vascular accident, 2 years ago, and was paralyzed on the right side of her upper body. She is obese (BMI 31), but does not like to do any exercise and has refused to participate in physical therapy. She spends most of the day in her apartment. After surgery, her pain is well controlled, and she began to walk using the rolling walker, but requires frequent reminders to ambulate. She is advised to take more fluids. However, she does not drink as much as she should, because she is worried about going to the bathroom so often. The nurse explained to her that hydration, exercise and proper nutrition are important measures to prevent thromboembolism after surgery. Nevertheless, she has not changed her behavior and continues to have a poor intake of fluids, and only ambulates when the nurse or physical therapist come into her room and have her walk.

Mrs. E.K.'s nursing diagnosis, key goals and outcomes, and general interventions

Nursing diagnosis	Risk for venous thromboembolism
Risk factors	• Dehydration • Impaired mobility • Obesity
Ultimate goal	Prevent venous thromboembolism
Key outcomes	▪ Appropriate hydration ▪ Appropriate exercise ▪ Appropriate amount and content of nutritional intake
General interventions	▪ Reinforce understanding of the importance of hydration ▪ Encourage to increase exercise ▪ Work with patient to develop a healthy nutritional plan she can implement at home

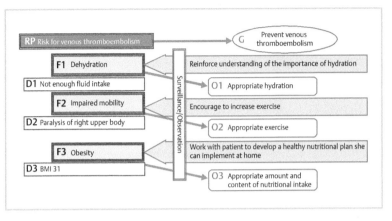

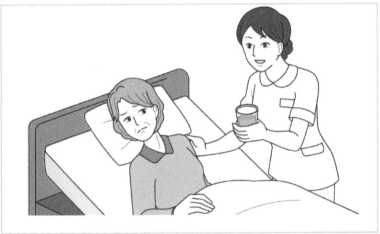

► Author's note ◄

This diagnosis was approved before NANDA-I introduced two new categories to the terminology, *at-risk populations* and *associated conditions*. Most of the suggested original risk factors are now found under these two categories. Current risk factors, impaired mobility and obesity, are not something that can be treated easily or quickly by the nurse. We would like to encourage further development of this diagnosis.

Domain 11. Safety/protection   Class 3. Violence
00272

Risk for Female Genital Mutilation

☞ *NANDA International Nursing Diagnoses: Definitions and Classification, 2018–2020,* p. 415

Definition

Susceptible to full or partial ablation of the female external genitalia and other lesions of the genitalia, whether for cultural, religious, or any other nontherapeutic reasons, which may compromise health.

Model case

Ms. M.T. is a 13-year-old immigrant from Africa. Her parents brought her and three younger siblings to the country 5 years earlier, as a result of war and famine. Her family lives in a community that includes a large number of African refugees, and where women's roles are very traditional. When she comes for a routine clinic visit, her mother seems to be very anxious about her reproductive health. She notes that she is undergoing puberty, and says she is worried about her daughter's fertility. When the nurse asks why she is concerned, her mother says that her daughter has not been "cut," and that it is "known" that an uncut clitoris leads to decreased fertility rates. She tells the nurse that her father is very worried that she will be considered undesirable for marriage unless she undergoes the procedure. He wants to find a local person to perform the ritual as soon as possible. However, Ms. M.T. makes it clear to the nurse that she does not want and does not consent to the female genital mutilation (FGM) ritual, and does not believe it is safe. The nurse recognizes that her mother believes a cultural myth that FGM increases fertility, and that her father believes it is important for his daughter.

M.T.'s nursing diagnosis, key goals and outcomes, and general interventions

Nursing diagnosis	Risk for female genital mutilation
Risk factors	• Lack of family knowledge about impact of practice on physical health • Lack of family knowledge about impact of practice on reproductive health • Lack of family knowledge about impact of practice on psycho-social health
Ultimate goal	Avoidance of female genital mutilation (FGM)
Key outcomes	• Improved parents' understanding of potential negative outcomes of FGM • Positive family relationship • Positive family support • Secured safety of Ms. M.T.
General interventions	• Provide parents with factual information on negative impacts of FGM • Provide support to parents as they consider their culturally held beliefs in light of new information provided • Consider community-based initiatives, including group meetings with community leaders, multimedia communications, and action plans to advocacy efforts • Consider inclusion of religious leaders in the community to facilitate greater knowledge uptake • Provide Ms. M.T. with support, emergency contacts, and protection if she feels she is at risk for FGM

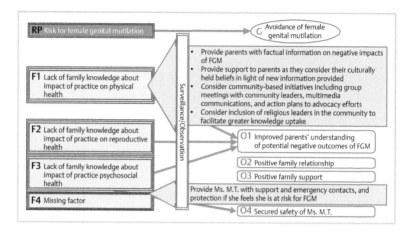

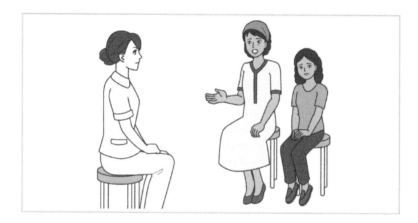

► Author's note ◄

Female genital mutilation is recognized internationally as a violation of the human rights of girls and women. Due to the complex nature of the phenomena, it is not easy to simplify relationships among the diagnosis, outcomes, and interventions. This diagnosis is classified under Domain 11 Safety/protection, Class 3 Violence; therefore, securing safety of Ms. M.T. is a crucial outcome. However, there is no corresponding risk factor. We would like to encourage further development of this diagnosis.

Domain 11. Safety/protection   Class 4. Environmental hazards
00265

Risk for Occupational Injury

☞ *NANDA International Nursing Diagnoses: Definitions and Classification, 2018–2020*, p. 427

Definition

Susceptible to a work-related accident or illness, which may compromise health.

Model case

Mr. N.T., 59 years old, works rotating 12-hour shifts at the industrial waste disposal plant. He comes to the clinic with complaints of insomnia and fatigue. All routine blood test results are normal. He does not have a good appetite, but he tries to eat properly to keep up his strength. He lost his previous job as a truck driver when his company went out of business. He had trouble finding similar work, so he reluctantly took the current job. He is not happy in this role, and he finds the environment very stressful. He thinks that he did not receive enough job training from his supervisor to handle possible biological and chemical hazards. He and his coworkers sometimes do not have the required protective equipment. He also feels protective equipment is uncomfortable and cumbersome, and sometimes does not use it even when it is available. His plant has been very busy, and always has a shortage of manpower, so he sometimes needs to work night shifts.

Mr. N.T.'s nursing diagnosis, key goals and outcomes, and general interventions

Nursing diagnosis	Risk for occupational injury
Risk factors	• Excessive stress • Improper use of personal protective equipment • Insufficient knowledge • Exposure to biological agents • Exposure to chemical agents • Night shift work rotating to day shift work
Ultimate goal	Free from occupational injury
Key outcomes	• Reduced stress • Proper use of protective equipment • Adequate knowledge to handle hazardous material • Adequate rest
General interventions	• Provide support to identify stress reduction methods • Ensure knowledge of the importance of protective equipment • Ensure knowledge of safe handling of hazardous material • Work with patient to identify a variety of methods to improve sleep

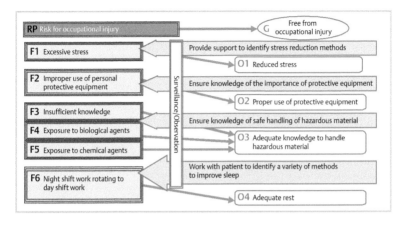

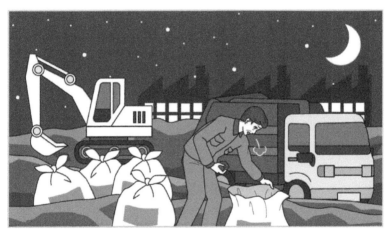

Domain 11. Safety/protection   Class 6. Thermoregulation
00274

Risk for Ineffective Thermoregulation

☞ *NANDA International Nursing Diagnoses: Definitions and Classification, 2018–2020,* p. 440

Definition

Susceptible to temperature fluctuation between hypothermia and hyperthermia, which may compromise health.

Model case

Mr. K.M., 76 years old, has been living in a skilled nursing home since his sister died 6 months ago. He had a spinal cord injury 10 years ago from an automobile accident; as a result, he relies on a wheelchair for mobility. He also has thermoregulation issues, which he has dealt with by means of frequent regulation of room temperature and dressing in appropriate clothing. During the regular clinic visit, he told the nurse that adjusting room temperature is very difficult this winter due to the facility's old heating system; his bedroom temperature is very different from that in the dining room and other shared spaces. This makes it difficult for him to select appropriate clothing, and he feels he is a burden to the staff to request help changing clothes or adding/removing blankets as the temperature changes. The environmental service manager has called the heating/air conditioning company to fix the problem, but they have been told it could be at least two weeks to get the necessary mechanical parts. He is very concerned that something may happen to his temperature while he sleeps.

Mr. K.M.'s nursing diagnosis, key goals and outcomes, and general interventions

Nursing diagnosis	Risk for ineffective thermoregulation
Risk factors	• Fluctuating environmental temperature
	• Inappropriate clothing for environmental temperature
	• Inactivity
Ultimate goal	Effective thermoregulation
Key outcomes	• Well managed environmental temperature
	• Appropriate clothing for environmental temperature
	• Appropriate activity

(Continued)

(Continued)

General interventions
- Adjust environmental temperature to the appropriate temperature
- Wear appropriate clothing for environmental temperature
- Have blankets available to address changing room temperatures
- Hourly rounding to check room and patient's temperature
- Work with environmental service staff to set alarm for temperature
  fluctuation in room of > 2 degrees

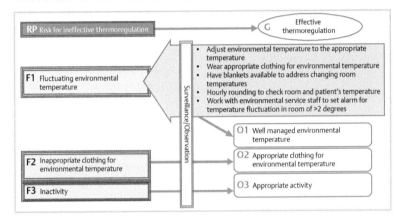

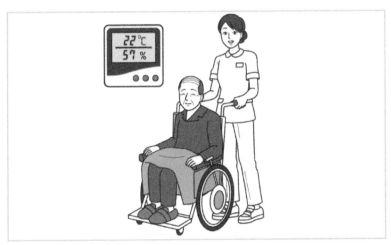

Bibliography

- Moorhead S, Johnson M, Maas ML, Swanson E. Nursing Outcomes Classification (NOC): Measurement of Health Outcomes [eBook]. 6th ed. St. Louis, MO: Elsevier; 2018
- Kim HS. The Nature of Theoretical Thinking in Nursing. 2nd ed. New York, NY: Springer; 2003
- Gordon M. Nursing Diagnosis: Process and Application. 3rd ed. St. Louis, MO: Mosby; 1994
- Kamitsuru S. Kangoshindankaramichibiku mokuhyoutokainyu model jitsu-zaigatashindandenokensyotosyusei [Outcome and intervention inference model for actual nursing diagnosis: validation and modification]. J Jpn Soc Nurs Diagn 2009; 14(2):166–167